Connected Health Insights for Sustainable Development

Shama Siddiqui • Anwar Ahmed Khan
Muazzam Ali Khan Khattak • Raazia Sosan

Connected Health Insights for Sustainable Development

Integrating IoT, AI, and Data-Driven Solutions

Springer

Shama Siddiqui
DHA Suffa University
Karachi, Pakistan

Muazzam Ali Khan Khattak
Quaid e Azam University
Islamabad, Pakistan

Anwar Ahmed Khan
Millennium Institute of Technology and Entrepreneurship
Karachi, Pakistan

Raazia Sosan
Salim Habib University
Karachi, Pakistan

ISBN 978-3-031-81432-7 ISBN 978-3-031-81433-4 (eBook)
https://doi.org/10.1007/978-3-031-81433-4

This Springer imprint is published by the registered company Springer Nature Switzerland AG
The registered company address is: Gewerbestrasse 11, 6330 Cham, Switzerland

Preface

Achieving sustainability is a dream of everyone. People plan for sustainability through setting personal goals, milestones. However, addressing global challenges requires a more complex approach to developing goals and milestones. The United Nations (UN) has tackled this complexity by creating the Sustainable Development Goals (SDGs), a comprehensive framework designed to address the world's most pressing issues. The 17 goals cover a broad spectrum of areas, including poverty, inequality, climate change, education, environment, and health, with SDG 3 specifically focusing on "Good Health and Well-Being" for all at all ages. The UN expects nations and individuals to work collaboratively toward achieving the SDGs by 2030. This requires a multifaceted approach where governments, private sectors, civil societies, and individuals must play critical roles.

Government all across the globe are striving to contribute to SDGs by taking diverse approaches. Various fundings have been made available, targeting specific SDGs and encouraging individuals and organization to pitch in their efforts. SDG 3 has been a key target area particularly for developing and under-developed regions where mostly lack of access to healthcare facilities is a major cause of high mortality. Some of the strategies developed to achieve SDG 3 include developing health infrastructure, investing in health workforce, managing nutrition and food security, developing/revising/implementing health policies and regulations, conducting public health programs, ensuring environmental health, and encouraging research and development. Using advanced information technology has also become a global norm for improving healthcare access, creating personalized healthcare service, and managing population health.

The next-generation technologies of Internet of Things (IoT), Data Science (DS), and Artificial Intelligence (AI) are expected to revolutionize the healthcare operation. Using these technologies, the patients can connect to the doctors and emergency service providers from anywhere, anytime; they can monitor their health trends right on their mobile applications and can also receive alerts about potential risks for their chronic diseases. Moreover, the governments can get detailed insights into population health trends, the probability of disease outbreaks, and future needs of resources. Based on these analytics, the policymakers are enabled for managing emergencies as well as for conducting routine awareness, training, and prevention programs to support health and well-being for their citizens.

We have designed this book to present the role of IoT, DS, and AI toward the global healthcare sector. We have dedicated a couple of chapters to explain the SDGs and fundamentals of IoT, DS, and AI technologies to provide a solid background for from diverse fields, including both computer scientists and social scientists. We have proposed IoT-DS-AI nexus that takes data from the users/patients using various forms of devices and apps, performs advanced analytics, and provides predictions. The advanced tools and techniques from each domain of this nexus would ensure effective individual and population health management.

From Chap. 3 onwards, we have described the detailed foundations, implementation, and challenges for IoT-DS-AI nexus for various healthcare applications. These include continuous health monitoring, m-Health and personalized medicine, digital imaging, population health surveillance, and resource optimization. In the end, we have presented overall challenges and opportunities for implementing the proposed technology nexus for achieving SDG 3.

Karachi, Pakistan — Shama Siddiqui
Karachi, Pakistan — Anwar Ahmed Khan
Islamabad, Pakistan — Muazzam Ali Khan Khattak
Karachi, Pakistan — Raazia Sosan

Contents

Chapter 1
Pioneering Health Technologies for Sustainable Development

1.1 What Are SDGs?

On September 25, 2015, the United Nations (UN) adopted the 2030 Agenda for Sustainable Development, which includes 17 Sustainable Development Goals (SDGs) aimed at addressing global challenges such as poverty, inequality, climate change, and peace and justice. The focus of SDGs is to achieve global sustainability and improved quality of life by 2030, through balancing economic, environmental and societal aspects; this 2030 agenda promises that "no one will be left behind" [1]. The SDGs are interwoven in such a way that achieving any one would have a lasting impact on the others. For example, reducing social inequalities is only possible by ensuring quality education, safe drinking water, and affordable healthcare for all. From all over the world, 193 countries (all members of the United Nations) have committed to work towards achieving this global sustainability agenda through developing cross-border strategies [2]. SDGs can be thought of as a comprehensive guidance framework for individuals, businesses and governments to work together in order to build a sustainable future. In this context, digital technologies can play a crucial role for the achievement of each SDG.

Prior to SDGs, UN had developed Millennium Development Goals (MDGs) in 2000, that were expired in 2015. The MDGs focused on reducing extreme poverty and improving basic health and education, whereas the SDGs expand the agenda to include a wider array of global challenges and set more ambitious targets [3]. SDGs have a much wider scope by addressing issues such as economic inequality, sustainable development, and stronger governance, which were not addressed earlier. Let's look at the evolution of SDGs as implemented by the UN.

S. Siddiqui et al., *Connected Health Insights for Sustainable Development*,
https://doi.org/10.1007/978-3-031-81433-4_1

1.2 History and Evolution: SDGs Versus MDGs

Just like SDGs, MDGs were also developed by the UN to address the most pressing global challenges through offering a guidance framework. The MDGs comprised eight specific targets aimed primarily at reducing extreme poverty and improving basic health and education outcomes [4]. These goals included eradicating extreme poverty and hunger, achieving universal primary education, promoting gender equality, reducing child mortality, improving maternal health, combating HIV/AIDS, malaria, and other diseases, ensuring environmental sustainability, and developing a global partnership for development.

The MDGs were instrumental in directing international efforts and resources towards addressing some of the most critical challenges faced by developing countries; these provided a clear and concise framework that allowed for measurable progress and accountability. As a result, significant strides were made in reducing the proportion of people living in extreme poverty, increasing primary school enrollment rates, and improving health outcomes, such as reductions in child mortality and the incidence of infectious diseases. However, the MDGs also faced criticisms and limitations: they were often considered too narrow in scope, as they focused primarily on the symptoms of poverty rather than its underlying causes. Additionally, the goals did not adequately address issues such as economic inequality, sustainable development, and the need for stronger institutions and governance.

In response to the above-described critiques and to build on the progress made by the MDGs, the UN introduced SDGs in 2015. The SDGs consist of 17 goals with 169 targets, encompassing a broader range of global challenges. These include not only the continuation of efforts to eradicate poverty and hunger but also the promotion of sustainable economic growth, decent work for all, innovation, infrastructure development, and the reduction of inequalities within and among countries.

In contrast to the MDGs, SDGs place a stronger emphasis on environmental sustainability, addressing climate change, conserving natural resources, and protecting biodiversity. They also highlight the importance of peace, justice, and strong institutions, recognizing that sustainable development cannot be achieved without inclusive and accountable governance [5]. Furthermore, the SDGs advocate for a holistic and integrated approach to development, acknowledging the interconnectedness of social, economic, and environmental dimensions. They aim to leave no one behind, ensuring that the benefits of development are shared equitably among all people, particularly the most vulnerable and marginalized populations.

In addition, the SDGs also recognize the vital role of technology, innovation, and global partnerships in achieving these ambitious targets. SDGs regards it mandatory to have collaborative efforts between governments, the private sector, civil society, and international organizations to mobilize resources, share knowledge, and foster sustainable development practices worldwide.

While the MDGs focused on immediate needs such as reducing extreme poverty, hunger, and improving basic health and education, the SDGs propose a more comprehensive and long-term approach. The MDGs targeted urgent issues that directly affected the poorest populations, laying the foundation for human development. In contrast, the SDGs address a broader range of global challenges, including inequality, climate change, and environmental sustainability [6]. They emphasize reducing inequalities, protecting ecosystems, promoting responsible consumption, and ensuring inclusive economic growth. Additionally, the SDGs highlight the importance of strong institutions, peace, and justice as essential components of sustainable development.

There has been a consistent review mechanism to audit the status of SDG achievement globally. Every year, the UN Secretary General delivers an annual SDG Progress report, created in collaboration with the UN System. This report is based on the global indicator framework and utilizes data produced by national statistical systems and information gathered at the regional level.

1.3 Sustainable Development Goals (SDGs): An Overview

The 17 SDGs outlined by United Nations are listed in Fig. 1.1. These goals are developed after identifying the most critical global challenges and announced as a global call for action. By developing the SDGs, United Nations has provided an opportunity for different sectors, countries and agencies to come together and work towards achieving sustainability [7]. All goals are closely linked to each other, with the overall objective of reducing inequalities and, improving peace, quality of life and health; the goals have to be achieved by ensuring innovation in technology development, policy making, sustainable practices, global partnerships, and active engagement of all stakeholders, including governments, private sector, civil society, and local communities.

SDGs provide a comprehensive framework to tackle the major global issues in an integrated way; these include poverty, hunger, inequality, climate change, and environmental degradation. Each Sustainable SDG has been strategically defined with key targets and implementation strategies to ensure measurable progress and

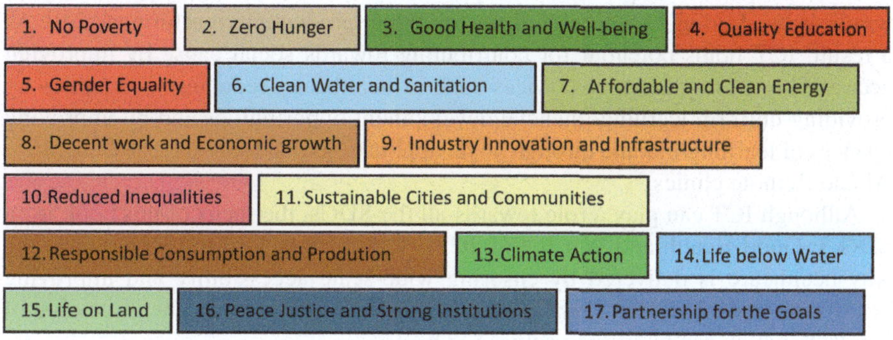

Fig. 1.1 17 SDGs by United Nations [7]

accountability. The designed targets outline specific, actionable steps that countries and stakeholders must take to achieve the overarching goals. For example, SDG 1 aims to end poverty in all its forms everywhere by targeting areas such as social protection systems, equal rights to economic resources, and resilience to environmental, economic, and social shocks. Similarly, SDG 13 focuses on combating climate change and its impacts through targets that promote climate resilience, improve education and awareness, and integrate climate change measures into national policies. Implementation strategies for each SDG emphasize the need for multi-stakeholder partnerships, adequate financing, technology transfer, capacity-building, and inclusive governance frameworks. This structured approach ensures that the SDGs are not only aspirational but also actionable, providing a clear roadmap for sustainable development efforts worldwide.

1.4 Technology and SDGs

For implementation of the 2030 agenda, Technology, science and capacity building have been identified as the major pillars. The environmentally sound technologies are very closely associated with the means of implementation for each SDG through innovation, business development, trade finance and capacity building [8]. Some of the common technologies, along with their contributions towards SDGs are presented in Fig. 1.2.

Information and Communication Technology (ICT) can particularly help to achieve each of the above-mentioned SDGs. Table 1.1 lists some of the ways in which ICT can contribute to achieve each SGD.

The emerging ICTs can address a wide range of global challenges ranging from individual health to global climate change. The major facility offered by ICT is internet connectivity, which provides access to data of any sector, to anywhere, any time. If we look closely at the ICT contributions listed in Table 1.1, it is evident that all SDGs are supported by means of data generation, sharing, storage or analytics. Secondly, there have been rapid advancements in the sectors of IoT, AI and data science, which further provides an opportunity to analyze the collected data in unique ways, leading to helpful insights and better productivity/performance [9]. As a result, ICT holds potential for contributing towards social cause by improving accessibility to fundamental services such as healthcare, reducing inequalities by providing uniform learning/financial/development opportunities and by improving chances of learning/income through novel applications and tools such as Generative AI and Remote clinics.

Although ICT can play a role towards all the SDGs, the focus of this book is on SDG 3: Good Health and Wel Being. ICTs hold the potential to revolutionize the way healthcare is delivered by ensuring wide-scale accessibility and improving health outcomes. Let's have a brief look at this SDG, followed by the discussion of key ICTs which can be used to achieve SDG 3.

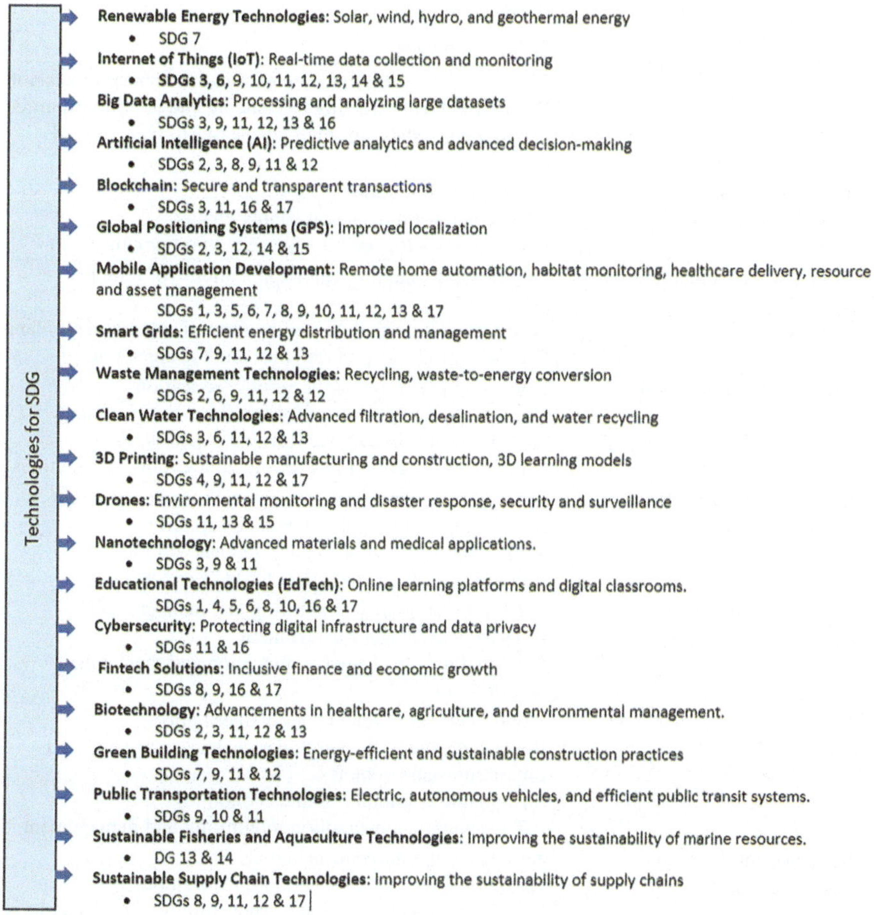

Fig. 1.2 Mapping between technologies to SDGs

1.5 What Is SDG 3?

The focus of SDG 3 is on ensuring health for all people of every age. UN has set well-defined targets to ensure access to quality healthcare services for everyone globally. The key targets and indicators of SDG3 are illustrated in Fig. 1.3 and discussed below:

1.6 Key Targets of SDG 3

The following targets are set to be achieved by 2030:

- Target 3.1: Maternal Mortality

Table 1.1 Ways in which ICT support SDGs

SDG	ICT contribution
SDG 1: No Poverty	Mobile banking and fintech solutions for financial inclusion Digital platforms creating freelancing and job opportunities. E-commerce enabling small businesses to reach global markets
SDG 2: Zero Hunger	Precision farming using IoT sensors and drones. Blockchain for transparent supply chains Data analytics for optimizing agricultural practices
SDG 3: Good Health and Well-being	Telemedicine and m-Health applications for remote healthcare AI for predictive analytics and personalized treatment plans Big data for disease surveillance and management
SDG 4: Quality Education	E-learning platforms for accessible education Developing digital skillset for futuristic career options AR and VR for immersive learning experiences Online collaboration tools for global learning communities
SDG 5: Gender Equality	Digital literacy programs for women's empowerment Mobile apps for health, safety, and support Online platforms for advocacy and networking Promoting Female leadership for tech sectors
SDG 6: Clean Water and Sanitation	IoT for water quality monitoring and management ICTs for wastewater management Data analytics for resource allocation and managing consumption
SDG 7: Affordable and Clean Energy	Smart grids for efficient energy distribution Renewable energy technologies such as solar and wind Smart cities and vehicles Sustainable communities and economies IoT for energy consumption monitoring and management
SDG 8: Decent Work and Economic Growth	Job matching platforms using AI. Digital marketplaces for economic development Novel ICT based entrepreneurship ventures, for example, digital health and transportation apps. E-commerce for expanding business opportunities
SDG 9: Industry, Innovation, and Infrastructure	Improve the extent and quality of ICT infrastructure. IoT and AI for automated and secure industry infrastructure Blockchain for secure and transparent transactions Cloud computing for scalable and collaborative innovation hubs
SDG 10: Reduced Inequality	Assistive technologies for physically challenged people. Extending digital platforms for economic and educational inclusion Online advocacy for marginalized communities

(continued)

Table 1.1 (continued)

SDG	ICT contribution
SDG 11: Sustainable Cities and Communities	Urban planning using GIS and AI Smart public transit systems IoT for monitoring and managing urban infrastructure
SDG 12: Responsible Consumption and Production	Advanced recycling and waste management technologies Blockchain for transparent supply chains Data analytics for sustainable production and waste management practices
SDG 13: Climate Action	Green technologies for emission reduction Modeling using Digital Twin technologies. Satellite and AI for climate monitoring IoT and big data analytics for tracking environmental impacts
SDG 14: Life Below Water	Marine drones and sensors for monitoring ocean health Blockchain for sustainable fisheries IoT for pollution detection and management IoT for protection of endangered animals such as Dolphins Smart Buoys for remote monitoring of sea environment
SDG 15: Life on Land	Remote sensing for forest and wildlife monitoring Precision farming for sustainable agriculture GIS for land use planning and conservation IoT for protection of endangered animals such as Tigers and Elephants
SDG 16: Peace, Justice, and Strong Institutions	E-government for better relationship between state and citizens Blockchain for transparent governance AI and big data for improving legal processes. Digital platforms for citizen engagement and participation
SDG 17: Partnerships for the Goals	Digital collaboration tools for multi-stakeholder partnerships Cloud computing for shared data and resources Online platforms for tracking and reporting SDG progress

- The global maternal mortality ratio is to be reduced to less than 70 per 100, 000 live births.
- Target 3.2: Neonatal and Child Mortality
- For newborn children, the mortality ratio is to be reduced to at least 12 per 1000 live births. Also, mortality rates for the children under 5 is to be reduced to as low as 25 per 1000 live births.
- Target 3.3: Infectious Diseases
- The epidemics of AIDS, tuberculosis, malaria are to be ended. Moreover, the prevention also has to be ensured for neglected tropical diseases, combat hepatitis, waterborne diseases and other communicable diseases.
- Target 3.4: Noncommunicable Diseases
- Non-communicable diseases need to be prevented and treated in order to reduce by one third premature mortality.
- Target 3.5: Substance Abuse

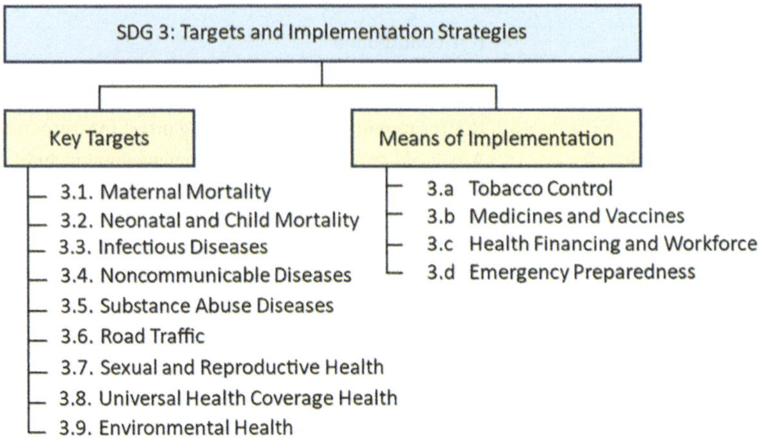

Fig. 1.3 Achieving SDG 3

- The substance abuse, including alcohol and narcotics, needs to be prevented and treated.
- Target 3.6: Road Traffic
- The number of global deaths happening due to road traffic accidents needs to be reduced by 50%.
- Target 3.7: Sexual and Reproductive Health
- The agenda of reproductive health shall be included into national strategies and programs for all countries. In addition, access to sexual and reproductive healthcare services will be ensured for everyone.
- Target 3.8: Universal Health Coverage
- Access to quality and affordable healthcare services, vaccines, and essential medicines will be ensured for everyone.
- Target 3.9: Environmental Health
- The number of deaths caused by environmental hazards such as air, soil and water pollution need to be substantially reduced.

1.7 Means of Implementation for SDG 3 Targets

The following means of implementation have been designed to achieve the above-listed targets of SDG 3.

- 3.a: Tobacco Control
- The WHO framework for Tobacco control needs to be implemented across all the countries.
- 3.b: Medicines and vaccines

- Medicines and vaccines need to be developed primarily for the communicable and non-communicable diseases that affect developing countries. Access to essential medicine and vaccines needs to be ensured for everyone in accordance with the guidelines offered by Doha Declaration on TRIPS and Public Health [10]; this declaration holds the right of developing countries to fully utilize the provisions in the Agreement on Trade-Related Aspects of Intellectual Property Rights (TRIPS agreement) to protect public health. Specifically, it emphasizes their ability to ensure access to medicines for all.
- 3.c: Health financing and workforce
- Health financing and recruitment need to be improved by a great deal for the developing, least developed and small island countries. There is not only a need to enhance training and development initiatives, but addressing the key challenge of health staff retention is also included in the implementation means.
- 3.d: Emergency preparedness

- The capacity of all countries, particularly, developing needs to be improved in terms of early warning, risk reduction and management of national and global health risks.

1.8 Internet of Things (IoT), Artificial Intelligence (AI) and Data Science (DS): Enabling Intelligent and Connected Health

Internet of Things (IoT) deals with using smart devices and sensors to collect and report real-time data for a wide variety of applications ranging from agriculture to healthcare. Data is collected periodically or on-demand and then communicated using conventional networking technologies such as 5G to the remote cloud servers [11]. From those servers, the data can be shared with interested stakeholders for remote monitoring, management of resources and data analytics. IoT has appeared as one of the major digital technologies to achieve SDGs through offering real-time data and insights. For example, IoT can provide agricultural data such as soil moisture level, humidity level and temperature to guide the farmers about optimal irrigation.

Data Science (DS) is an emerging field that works on scientific methods, processes, algorithms, and systems to extract knowledge and insights from structured and unstructured data. It is an interdisciplinary field which builds on the foundations of computer science, statistics, information theory and domain specific knowledge for analyzing and interpreting complex datasets. DS has been used in various industries for driving new insights from the data, leading to effective decision-making and process optimization [12]. Using advanced data analytics techniques, organizations become able to exploit their opportunities of exploring their environment and operations.

Artificial Intelligence (AI) is a transformative technology that enables machines to perform tasks that typically require human intelligence. AI systems can process large amounts of data, learn from it, and make decisions or predictions with minimal human intervention, using high computation power and advanced algorithms [13]. AI encompasses a wide range of subfields and applications, making it a versatile and powerful tool for nearly every domain: some sub-fields of AI include Machine Learning (ML), Natural Language Processing (NLP), Computer Vision, Robotics, Expert Systems and Reinforcement Learning.

The three technologies, IoT, Data Science and AI in fact, forms a nexus, termed as "IoT-DS-AI Nexus", as illustrated by Fig. 1.4. Data is generated and transmitted by the IoT devices which exist at the lowest level; it is stored and processed by data analytics algorithms existing at the middle level, and finally, trends and patterns in the data are identified using AI techniques that are present at the top level. These technologies along with their core concepts, will be discussed in detail, in the next chapter.

Using the above-described emerging technologies, can speed up progress on the 17 United Nations SDGs, as earlier indicated in Table 1.1. For example, all of these technologies may be used for upsurging the efficiency of urban industries, reducing the cost of urban services, increasing the productivity and competitiveness of the natural and human resources, and developing climate resilience [14]. However, SDG 3 can be regarded as the one most impacted; the application of these technologies in healthcare can lead to significant improvements in disease prevention, diagnosis, and treatment, ultimately enhancing the overall health and well-being of populations. For example, IoT solutions in healthcare track patient's data using wearable devices, monitor the health state remotely, connect with the remote

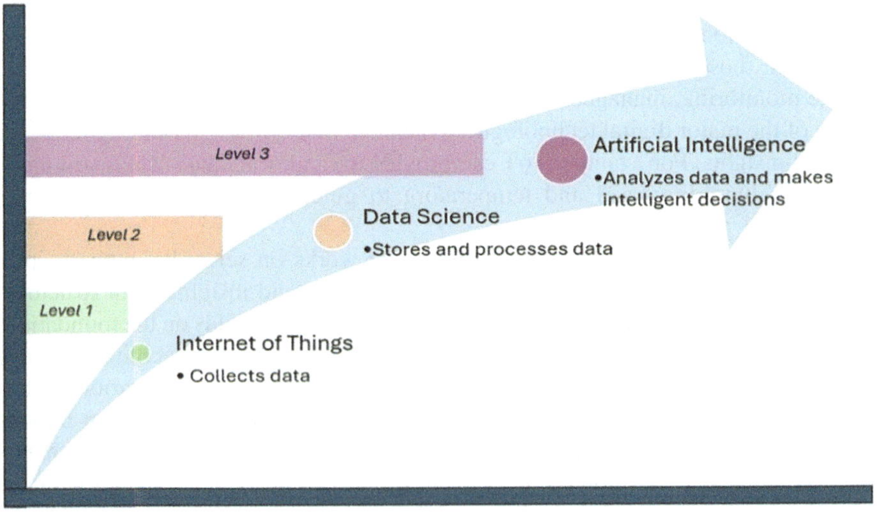

Fig. 1.4 IoT-DS-AI Nexus

physicians, maintain health records and deliver personalized and/or emergency services as needed. AI and Big data techniques can subsequently build on the data provided by IoT and can analyze large datasets to identify patterns, predict health trends, enhance diagnostic accuracy, and develop personalized treatment plans, thereby improving overall healthcare outcomes and efficiency [15].

1.9 Contents Overview

In this chapter, we set the foundation for the present book by providing details about SDGs and specifically SDG 3. The subsequent chapters are designed to describe each technology, IoT, DS and AI in their relation to SDGs. The contents are briefly described below:

Chapter 2 covers the fundamental concepts of IoT, AI and DS. It begins with an introduction to IoT, explaining its significance, components, architecture, applications, and the challenges it faces in driving sustainable development. The chapter then delves into AI, exploring its various branches, applications, ethical considerations, and future trends, all within the framework of contributing to SDGs. Following this, it introduces Data Science, discussing its key components, tools, applications, and associated challenges, emphasizing its role in data-driven decision-making for sustainable progress. The chapter concludes by highlighting the integration of IoT, AI, and Data Science, showcasing their synergies, practical case studies, and future directions, and demonstrating how these technologies collectively support the achievement of SDG 3.

The subsequent chapters deal with major applications supported by IoT, AI and DS as they have a direct contribution towards achieving SDG 3. Chapter 3 presents a detailed account on continuous monitoring which has been one of the major domains where IoT, ML and DS come into play. It highlights key applications such as wearable health devices, remote patient monitoring systems, and predictive analytics for early disease detection. The chapter also discusses the challenges and future trends in continuous monitoring, demonstrating how these technologies are crucial for enhancing public health and achieving the targets set by SDG 3.

Chapter 4 focuses on m-Health, and offers an insight into the use of mobile technologies for achieving SDG 3. Here, the history of m-Health is presented, followed by common categories and applications of m-Health apps. The emerging technologies supporting m-Health solutions and platforms have been discussed. By examining the integration of these technologies, the chapter illustrates how m-Health contributes to improved healthcare accessibility, efficiency, and quality. Therefore, this chapter demonstrates the transformative potential of mobile health technologies in driving progress towards the targets set by SDG 3, ultimately promoting healthier lives and well-being for all.

Chapter 5 has been designed to cover the aspect of personalized medicine which has become possible due to the integration of cutting-edge technologies of IoT, AI and DS. First, we describe the factors assessed for developing personalized medicine, such as genetic makeup, medical history, lifestyle, and environmental influences. These elements are critical in creating tailored healthcare solutions that meet individual patient needs. Subsequently, the deployment protocols of IoT, AI and DS for developing personalized medicines are presented, detailing how each is utilized to gather, analyze, and interpret patient data for personalized treatment plans. Hence, Chap. 5 highlights the profound impact of personalized medicine on patient outcomes and its significant role in advancing SDG 3.

Chapter 6 presents a detailed insight on how the conventional digital imaging techniques have been revolutionized using wearable/implantable sensing technologies, ML and Data Science. The chapter investigates the synergistic effects of these technologies, highlighting their collective impact on enhancing diagnostic accuracy, improving treatment outcomes, and fostering new avenues for research and development in healthcare and beyond. Ultimately, these advancements are aimed at contributing to the achievement of SDG 3.

Chapter 7 focuses on describing the role of IoT, DS and AI for fostering health surveillance among the population, and also, resource optimization which is a crucial need for governments. Here, we explore how these technologies enable real-time monitoring of health data, predictive analytics for disease outbreaks, and efficient allocation of resources. By using IoT, DS, and AI, governments can proactively address public health challenges, enhance surveillance capabilities, and optimize resource allocation strategies. These efforts aim to foster healthier populations and sustainable healthcare systems, aligning with the goals of SDG 3 to ensure healthy lives and promote well-being for all.

In Chap. 8, we conclude the book by addressing significant ethical considerations and implementation challenges associated with IoT, AI, and DS. This chapter explores the complexities of integrating these technologies into healthcare systems, highlighting ethical dilemmas and proposing strategies for responsible implementation. By navigating these challenges thoughtfully, stakeholders can work towards enhancing healthcare delivery and achieving SDG 3.

References

1. Valtioneuvoston kanslia, "Report on the Implementation of the 2030 Agenda for Sustainable Development," Voluntary National Review 2020 Finland, 2020
2. M. Mishra et al., A bibliometric analysis of sustainable development goals (SDGs): A review of progress, challenges, and opportunities. Environ. Dev. Sustain. **26**(5) (2024). https://doi.org/10.1007/s10668-023-03225-w
3. D. Mhlanga, A historical perspective on sustainable development and the sustainable development goals, in *FinTech and Artificial Intelligence for Sustainable Development*, Sustainable Development Goals Series, (Palgrave Macmillan, Cham, 2023). https://doi.org/10.1007/978-3-031-37776-1_4
4. J. Servaes, Introduction: From MDGs to SDGs, in *Sustainable Development Goals in the Asian Context*, (2017). https://doi.org/10.1007/978-981-10-2815-1_1

5. S. Kannengießer, From millennium development goals to sustainable development goals: Transforming development communication to sustainability communication. Stud. Commun. Sci. **23**(1) (2023). https://doi.org/10.24434/j.scoms.2023.01.3516
6. S. Arora-Jonsson, The sustainable development goals: A universalist promise for the future. Futures **146** (2023). https://doi.org/10.1016/j.futures.2022.103087
7. THE 17 GOALS | Sustainable Development. Accessed 01 Aug 2024. [Online]. Available: https://sdgs.un.org/goals
8. M. Al-Emran, C. Griffy-Brown, The role of technology adoption in sustainable development: Overview, opportunities, challenges, and future research agendas. Technol. Soc. **73** (2023). https://doi.org/10.1016/j.techsoc.2023.102240
9. J. Dzator, A.O. Acheampong, I. Appiah-Otoo, M. Dzator, Leveraging digital technology for development: Does ICT contribute to poverty reduction? Telecommun. Policy **47**(4) (2023). https://doi.org/10.1016/j.telpol.2023.102524
10. WTO | Ministerial conferences—Doha 4th Ministerial—TRIPS declaration. Accessed 01 Aug 2024. [Online]. Available: https://www.wto.org/english/thewto_e/minist_e/min01_e/mindecl_trips_e.htm
11. I. Rafiq, A. Mahmood, S. Razzaq, S.H.M. Jafri, I. Aziz, IoT applications and challenges in smart cities and services. J. Eng. **4**, 2023 (2023). https://doi.org/10.1049/tje2.12262
12. M. Nilashi, O. Keng Boon, G. Tan, B. Lin, R. Abumalloh, Critical data challenges in measuring the performance of sustainable development goals: Solutions and the role of big-data analytics. Harv. Data. Sci. Rev. **5**(3) (2023). https://doi.org/10.1162/99608f92.545db2cf
13. Z. Fan, Z. Yan, S. Wen, Deep learning and artificial intelligence in sustainability: A review of SDGs, renewable energy, and environmental health. Sustainability (Switzerland) **15**(18) (2023). https://doi.org/10.3390/su151813493
14. M. Arfanuzzaman, Harnessing artificial intelligence and big data for SDGs and prosperous urban future in South Asia. Environ. Sustain. Ind. **11** (2021). https://doi.org/10.1016/j.indic.2021.100127
15. D. Teh, T. Rana, The use of internet of things, big data analytics and artificial intelligence for attaining UN's SDGs, in *Handbook of Big Data and Analytics in Accounting and Auditing*, (2023). https://doi.org/10.1007/978-981-19-4460-4_11

Chapter 2
Fundamentals of Internet of Things (IoT), Artificial Intelligence (AI) and Data Science (DS)

2.1 Overview of IoT

IoT refers to a network of physical objects embedded with software and hardware, capable of sensing and transmitting data. The most common task of IoT devices is to send data over internet for remote monitoring and management of resources. Today (2024), the estimated number of IoT devices connected to internet is 17.02 billion and the number is estimated to reach 32.1 billion in 2030 [1]. However, the technology originated from the fundamental desire to connect and monitor remote objects; initially, a student at Carnegie Melon university wanted to know the status of soda machine that operated at his department. Subsequently, the objects such as toaster and coffee machines were connected, and today we have entire smart homes and healthcare facilities connected and operated over internet [2]. A brief timeline indicating evolution of IoT has been illustrated in Fig. 2.1.

Thus, starting with a connected vending machine in 1982, the trend of connecting things to internet followed by connected toasters and coffee machines in 1990 and 1993 respectively. The technology gained further traction in 1999 with the implementation of RFID for supply chain management. Significant milestones included the International Telecommunication Union's formal acknowledgment of IoT in 2005 and the first IoT conference held in 2008, marking a pivotal moment for the industry. By 2012, the integration of AI into personal assistants demonstrated the advanced capabilities of IoT systems, showcasing their growing sophistication and application in everyday technology.

Next, we describe the architecture and key components of IoT.

S. Siddiqui et al., *Connected Health Insights for Sustainable Development*,
https://doi.org/10.1007/978-3-031-81433-4_2

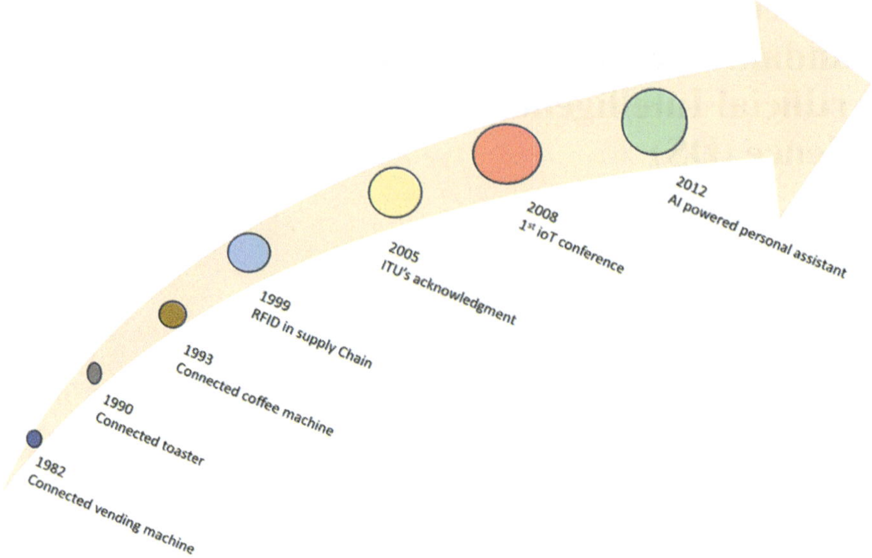

Fig. 2.1 Evolution of IoT

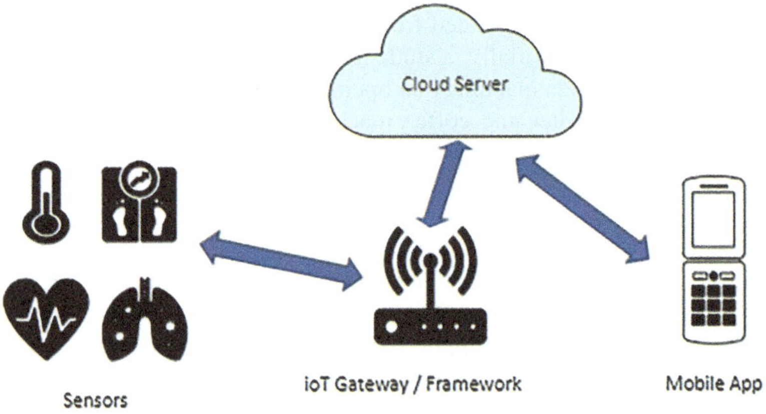

Fig. 2.2 Basic architecture of IoT

2.1.1 IoT Architecture

The most basic architecture of IoT, as applicable for most scenarios is illustrated in Fig. 2.2. At the foundation of all IoT solutions, there are sensing devices which could sense physical parameters such as temperature, humidity etc. The sensed data is transmitted using any communication technology such as Wi-Fi/4G/Bluetooth to the cloud servers; subsequently, the data can be accessed via diverse types of mobile apps and dashboards.

In terms of layers, IoT is generally defined as a three-layered architecture; it comprises of perception, network and application layers [3]. Each layer has distinct responsibilities but works together to collect, transmit, process, and utilize data. At the lowest level, perception Layer, also known as device or sensor layer, is responsible for data acquisition. It includes all the physical devices and sensors that gather data from the environment. At the middle level, network layer, also known as the communication layer, is responsible for transmitting the data collected by the perception layer to the next layer for processing. It handles the communication and connectivity aspects of the IoT system. Finally, the topmost layer is application, where data processing, analysis, and user interactions take place. It provides the end-user services and applications that make use of the collected data to deliver actionable insights and functionalities. The essential components of each layer are shown in Fig. 2.3.

2.1.2 Key Applications of IoT

Emerging IoT solutions can be deployed to serve a large number of public and private applications, of varying scales. For example, a person might locate their pet using RFID tag or a state official may look for the flood prone areas for disaster prevention, using ultrasonic sensors. A list of common IoT applications has been presented in Fig. 2.4. Since the focus of this book is on SDG 3, let's discuss IoT for healthcare in some detail.

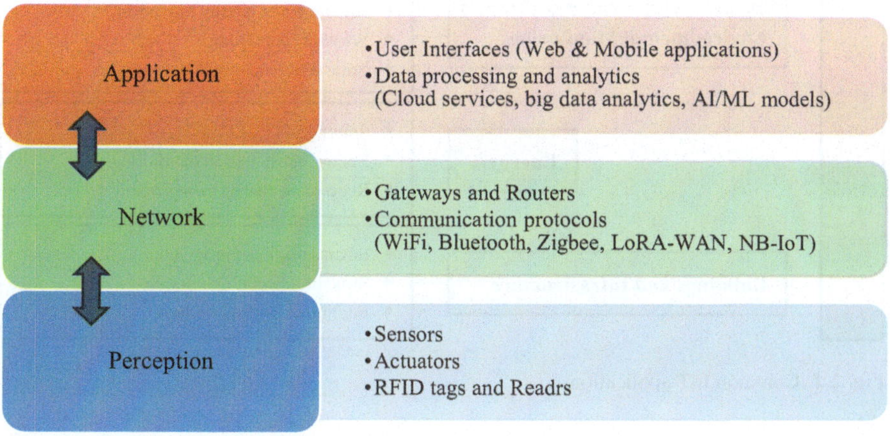

Fig. 2.3 Layered architecture of IoT

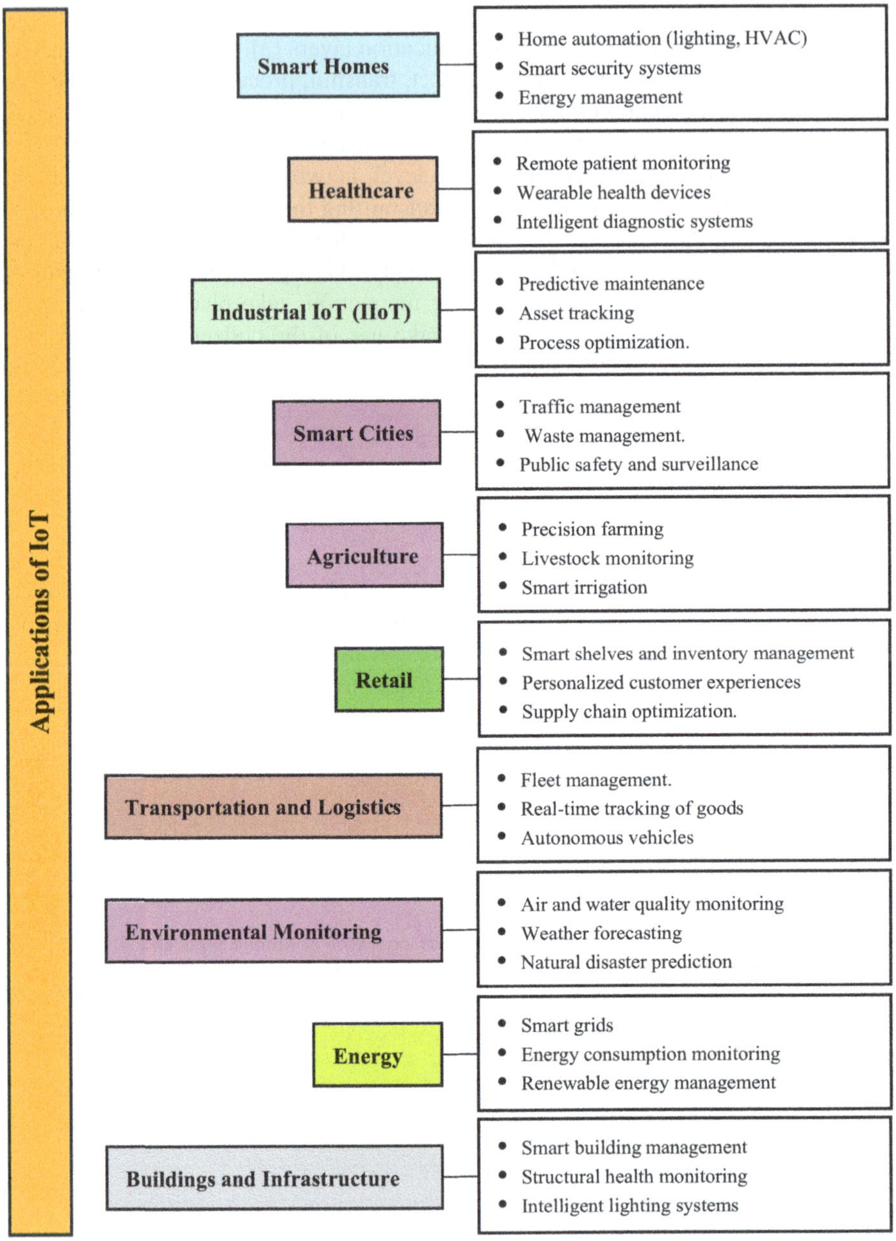

Fig. 2.4 Common IoT applications

2.1.3 IoT in Healthcare

The use of IoT for sensing and communicating has potential to revolutionize the healthcare sector. Fundamentally, use of IoT for health-related applications deal with continuous monitoring, real-time data collection, and intelligent diagnostics. The major drivers for the increasing use and acceptance of IoT for health include increasing cost of healthcare, low access to facilities for population, increasing elderly population with one or more chronic disease that needs continuous monitoring and the desire of patients and doctors for remote connectivity [4]. By integrating IoT into healthcare systems, we can enhance patient outcomes through timely interventions, reduce overall healthcare costs, and make healthcare services more accessible and efficient.

Some of the key benefits of IoT for the healthcare domain have been highlighted in Fig. 2.5. First and foremost, IoT solutions are used for remote monitoring of the patients for management of different chronic diseases, or simply for fitness monitoring. The healthcare become much more cost-effective and accessible due to the use of wearable and environmental IoT devices as the information continuously flows to the doctors and the need of physical clinical visit significantly reduces. The data about monitored vital parameters such as blood pressure, glucose levels, ECG, etc. is stored locally or online; this provides an opportunity of maintaining detailed health analytics which is not possible otherwise. The patients and doctors both benefit from the availability of customized health trends just by accessing already stored data; clearly, this feature of health IoT solutions help in early intervention as well as informed decision making. Earlier, patients often face the hassle of maintaining paper-based health records and presenting the same to their doctors; however, IoT makes this task easier through offering a large number of mobile apps and digital platforms.

Patient engagement and empowerment are also strongly affected with the help of IoT solutions. The apps mostly encourage the patients to regularly enter the data

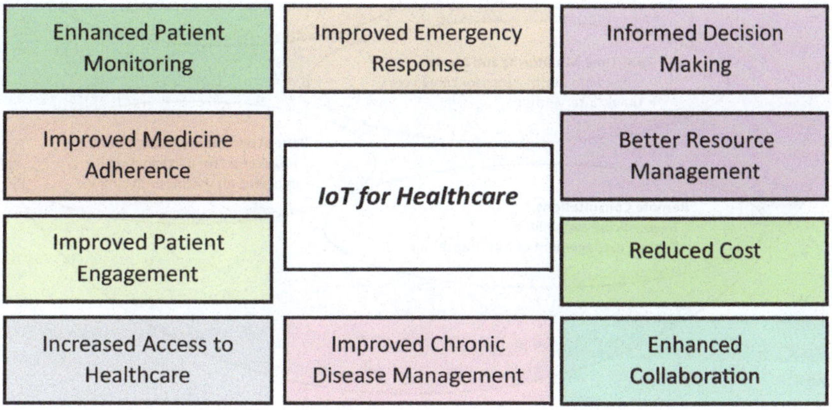

Fig. 2.5 Key benefits of IoT for healthcare

about their medication/diagnostic tests/fitness goals etc. Subsequently, the apps automatically send reminders about activities such as taking medicine, working out, visiting doctor and engage with community. Moreover, by looking at the health records and trends, the chronic patients feel more interested to maintain or improve their records. Also, by engaging with a community through these platforms, patients receive support and motivation from peers. Therefore, the continuous patient involvement realized due to IoT devices fosters a sense of control and responsibility, leading to better adherence to treatment plans and proactive health management.

Moreover, the emergency access to healthcare has also become a lot easier by virtue of IoT, as the doctors and emergency service providers are always connected. Data through patient wearable is continuously assessed and in case of elevated risk, the alerts are transmitted to the hospital for sending in the emergency support. The feature of emergency detection has gained a wide popularity in the countries having a large ratio of independently living elderly; a concept termed Ambient Assisted Living (AAL) has been coined [5], which refers to creating a smart environment that could assist the elderly in managing the emergency situations and also,

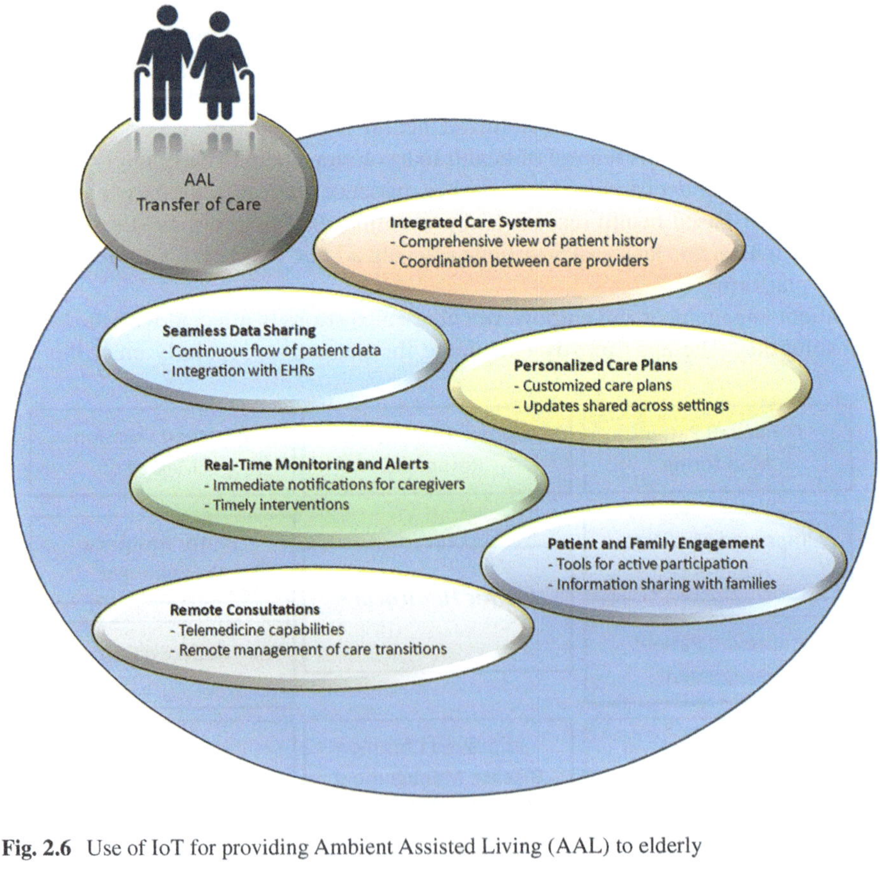

Fig. 2.6 Use of IoT for providing Ambient Assisted Living (AAL) to elderly

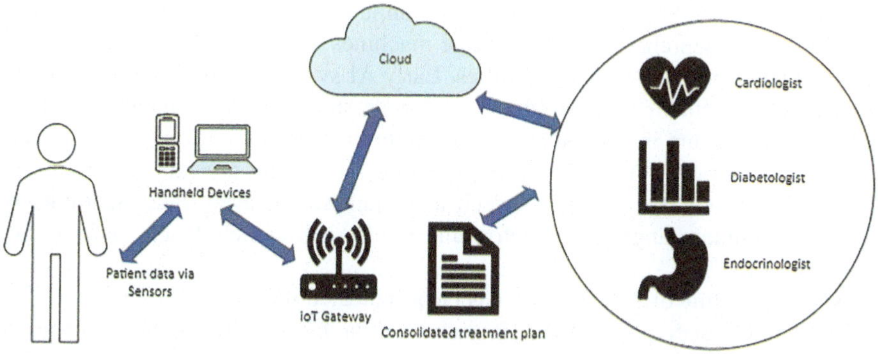

Fig. 2.7 Cardiology

completing their day-to-day tasks. A typical model for transfer of care using AAL is depicted in Fig. 2.6.

There are also several IoT benefits for the hospitals and state. The hospitals can efficiently plan their resources including equipment, wards and staff using the data collected from IoT sensors. Using various sensors and RFID tags, it becomes easy for the healthcare facilities to track the location of their staff and equipment. Also, based on the data about use, logs and health of equipment, the hospitals can engage in predictive maintenance of medical equipment, leading to reduced downtimes and increased rate of patient service and satisfaction. The collaboration among doctors and medical experts also become more practical and simpler using IoT solutions; the data can seamlessly flow from patients' wearables to multiple doctors who might be involved in the patients' treatment. As a result, all the experts can collaborate and reach a consensus about the diagnosis and personalized treatment plan for the patients. An example case of medical collaboration achieved using Health IoT has been illustrated in Fig. 2.7, where a patient may need constant assistance from multiple doctors including cardiologist, diabetologist and endocrinologist. Having access to patient data, all the doctors will ensure that no treatment strategy conflict takes place.

2.2 Overview of AI

Artificial Intelligence (AI) refers to the simulation of human intelligence in machines, enabling them to perform tasks that typically require human cognition, such as learning, reasoning, problem-solving, and decision-making. AI systems use algorithms and models to process large amounts of data, identify patterns, and make predictions or decisions based on that data. The most common application of AI is to enhance automation and improve efficiency across various industries. Today, AI technologies are integral to numerous applications, including virtual assistants, autonomous vehicles, and predictive analytics.

The concept of AI has its roots in early computer science and cognitive psychology. Initially, researchers aimed to create machines that could mimic basic human reasoning and problem-solving abilities. Early AI systems were developed to play games, solve mathematical problems, and understand natural language [6]. Over time, advancements in computing power, data availability, and algorithmic techniques have propelled AI to new heights. Today, AI systems are capable of learning from vast datasets, recognizing speech and images, and even understanding and generating human language, transforming fields such as healthcare, finance, and manufacturing.

A brief timeline of AI evolution has been indicated in Fig. 2.8.

In 1940, the decryption of the Enigma machine by Alan Turing and his team at Bletchley Park laid the groundwork for computational techniques foundational to AI. The 1950s saw Alan Turing introduce the Turing Test, a criterion for determining whether a machine can exhibit human-like intelligence, and in 1955, John McCarthy coined the term "Artificial Intelligence," formally inaugurating the field [6]. By 1961, the introduction of *Unimate*, the first industrial robot, signified the beginning of automation in manufacturing. In 1964, *Eliza*, the first chatbot created by Joseph Weizenbaum, was capable of simulating conversation with users, while in 1969, *Shakey*, developed by SRI International, became the first mobile robot capable of making decisions about its actions by perceiving its environment.

The 1990s and 2000s saw substantial advancements in AI. In 1995, *ALICE* (Artificial Linguistic Internet Computer Entity) showcased progress in natural

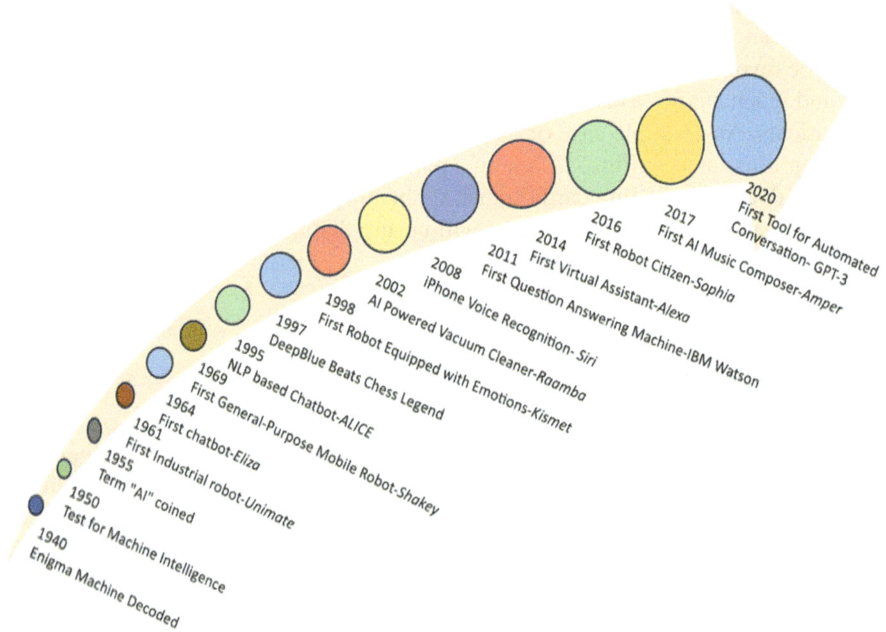

Fig. 2.8 AI evolution timeline

language processing. IBM's DeepBlue defeated world chess champion Garry Kasparov in 1997, marking a significant achievement. In 1998, MIT's *Kismet* became the first robot designed to recognize and simulate emotions. The early 2000s brought AI into everyday life with the 2002 launch of *Raamba*, an AI-powered vacuum cleaner by iRobot. The introduction of voice recognition on the iPhone in 2008 with Siri further integrated AI into consumer technology. In 2011, IBM Watson, the first question-answering machine, was developed. Amazon's *Alexa*, the first virtual assistant, was released in 2014, followed by the creation of *Sophia*, the first robot citizen, in 2016. The creative potential of AI was highlighted in 2017 with the introduction of Amper, the first AI music composer. The release of GPT-3 by OpenAI in 2020 represented a major leap in AI capabilities, providing a powerful tool for automated conversation and demonstrating the convergence of AI and Natural Language Processing.

2.2.1 Key Techniques of AI

The AI landscape encompasses a wide range of technologies and applications that enhance various aspects of human-computer interaction and data analysis. Some of these have been shown in Fig. 2.9:

Clearly, each emerging technology from the domain of AI has a potential to revolutionize the computing tasks. **Speech Recognition** technologies enable systems to interpret and respond to voice commands, provide transcription services, and authenticate users through voice biometrics. **Natural Language Processing (NLP)** involves text classification, sentiment analysis, machine translation, chatbots, virtual assistants, and named entity recognition, allowing systems to understand and generate human language effectively. **Computer Vision** technologies facilitate image classification, object detection, image segmentation, facial recognition, and optical character recognition (OCR), enabling machines to interpret and analyze visual information. **Predictive Analytics** is used for risk management, customer behavior prediction, demand forecasting, and fraud detection, helping organizations make data-driven decisions. **Recommendation Systems** personalize content, product recommendations, target marketing, and social media suggestions based on user preferences. Finally, **Robotic Process Automation (RPA)** streamlines workflow automation, data extraction, task automation, process optimization, and system integration, improving efficiency and productivity across various industries.

2.2.2 Key Applications of AI

The key applications of AI span across various industries, driving innovation and enhancing efficiency. From healthcare and finance to entertainment and transportation, AI technologies are transforming how businesses operate and how services are

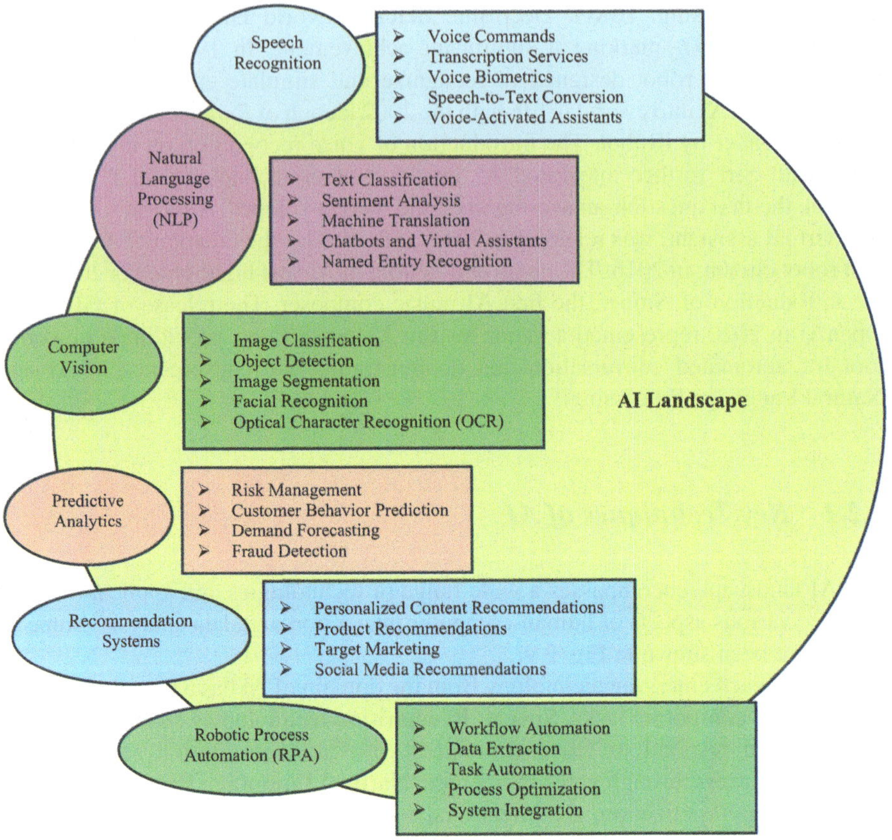

Fig. 2.9 Enabling technologies of AI

delivered. By leveraging advanced algorithms and data analysis, AI enables intelligent decision-making, automation, and personalized experiences, making it an indispensable tool in the modern world. Some of the key applications are listed in Fig. 2.10:

2.2.3 AI in Healthcare

AI has a diverse set of applications in healthcare; it has been used for robot-assisted surgeries, personalized medicine recommendations, health-trend analysis, genetic code analysis, etc. typically, the technologies of NLP, ML and DL have been used in healthcare. Over the past decade, AI has increasingly been used for performing the tasks that were done by human; by using predictive analytics and data processing capabilities of AI, the healthcare professionals can take a more proactive

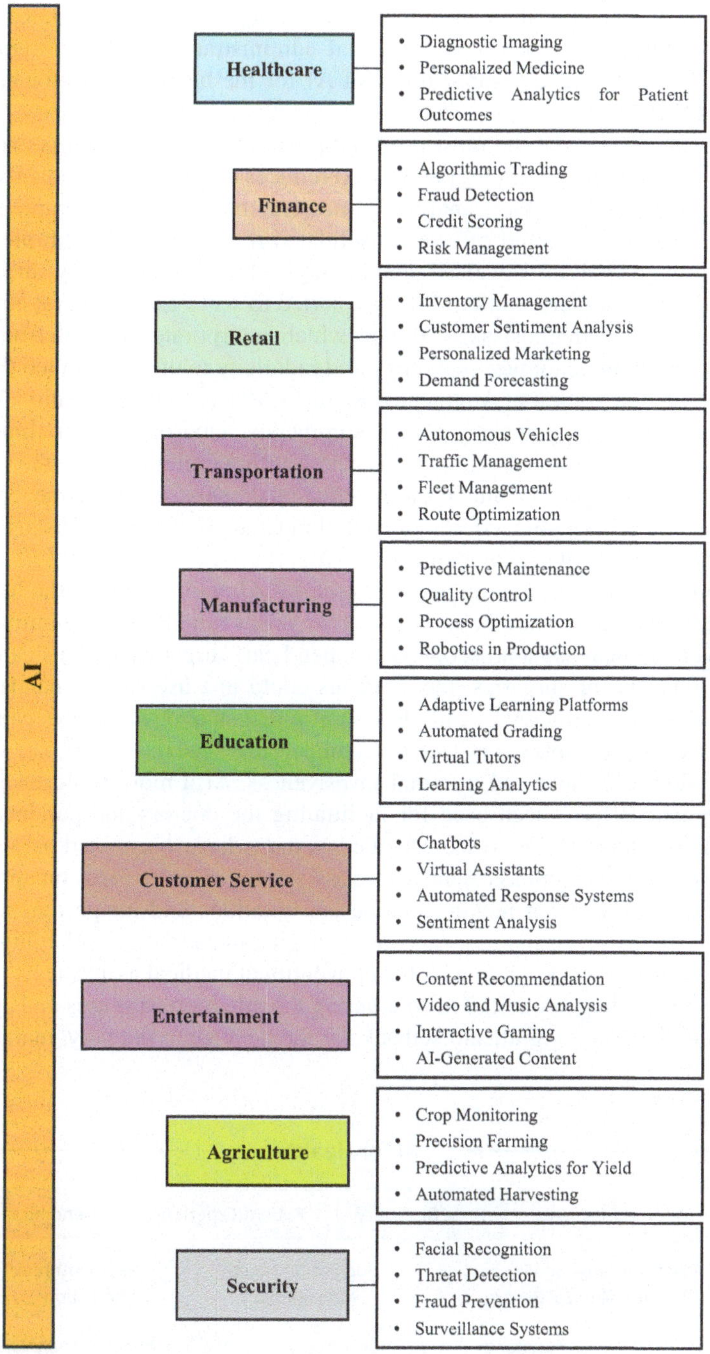

Fig. 2.10 Key applications of AI

approach for managing their resources and developing treatment strategies. As a result, the burden on doctors and hospital administrators has been significantly reduced. Some of the key applications of AI for the healthcare sector have been identified Fig. 2.11:

Diagnostics is one of the most promising applications of AI that is expected to reduce the preventable harm for patients. AI reduces the chance of medical errors by providing accurate and timely analysis of massive, distributed and complex medical data. For example, it could offer a consolidated response about multiple medical images through applying novel ML and DL algorithms, which clearly surpasses the human vision and interpretation. ML has started to serve as an integral component of computer-aided diagnosis (CAD) tools which incorporates the data from various domains including genomics, pathology and radiology to offer a detailed diagnosis. Similarly, the integration of Augmented Reality (AR) and Virtual Reality (VR) with AI for medical imaging analysis provides immersive environment for clinical practice as well as professional trainings [7]; these technologies enhance the visualization of medical images, leading to a more efficient diagnosis and treatment planning. This subject has been covered in more detail in Chap. 6, where we discuss cutting-edge techniques about digital medical imaging.

Robotic surgery was among one of the initial AI applications in the healthcare. Today, advanced robots are being used for surgeries ranging from minimally invasive surgeries (such as laparoscopies), to open heart surgeries. Robots can be used at various levels for surgeries; the surgeons could just use robot's hands for precisely performing surgeries, while they sit at a distance, or the robots can autonomously execute complex surgical tasks under the supervision of the surgeons, ensuring high precision and minimal invasiveness. At a more basic level, virtual health assistants have been used for facilitating the doctors and patients; mobile applications, chatbots and voice-activated systems have been used as a common example of virtual health assistant. These assistants generally focus on applications such as clinical decision making, online consultations and image diagnosis. The major advantage of virtual assistance is their guaranteed 24/7 availability/accessibility, which is never possible with the conventional medical assistance.

AI also has a huge potential for predicting the infectious diseases and epidemics [8]. Epidemics cause significant setback for the healthcare industry, mainly due to

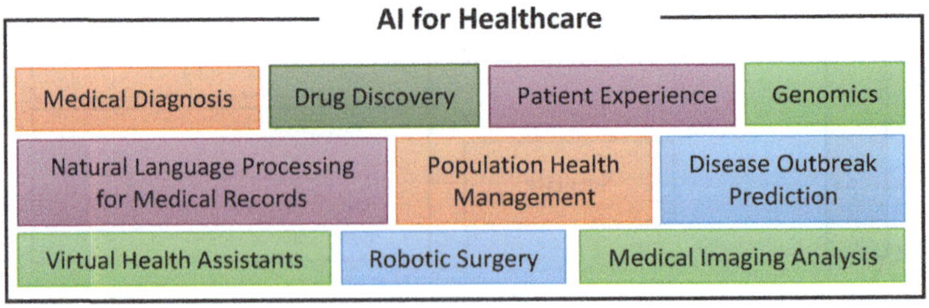

Fig. 2.11 Applications of AI

the resulting shortage of medicines, supplies, protective equipment, staff and facilities. Traditional epidemiological models developed during the early twentieth century have helped us understand disease spread. However, today's complex global interactions and vast amounts of data require more advanced predictive tools. AI uses real-time monitoring and data integration for precisely predicting the infectious diseases; the accuracy of AI algorithms is significantly better in contrast to the conventional models. This development brought by the AI is expected to particularly uplift the healthcare in the developing regions where it is highly likely to have large-scale disease outbreaks. Thus, the population health management is improved through efficient resource allocation and preventive strategy implementation.

Personalized medicine and predictive analytics gained a wide popularity due to the integration of modern computing technologies including AI. AI provides in-depth analysis into the patient's profile not only by providing comprehensive medical history, but also by performing detailed genetic analysis. Genome sequence is performed to aid in identifying the diseases which is not possible otherwise. Generative AI also enhances the capacity of AI models for data analysis and interpretation, facilitating various applications such as identification of biomarkers for drug discovery, analysis of EHR data, assessment of medical images and supporting clinical decisions [4]. Hence, the use of AI for personalized medicine would transform the healthcare because as proactive treatment strategies shall be implemented instead of the conventional reactive.

Drug discovery is another domain which has been influenced by AI. It is the process of identifying and developing new medicines, and conducting clinical trials before launching into the markets. It has been a very complex and costly process, which has been improved through the data processing and analytics capability of ML algorithms. For example, DL can be used for accurately identifying the efficacy of medical compounds, as well as to identify the best participants for clinical trials [9]. Moreover, AI techniques can also predict the toxic effects of medicines; particularly, based on the genetic analysis used in personalized medicine, it has become possible for the ML algorithms to identify the possible side effects of medicines for unique patient profiles.

2.3 Overview of DS

Data Science (DS) refers to the interdisciplinary field that uses scientific methods, processes, algorithms, and systems to extract knowledge and insights from structured and unstructured data. Data Science combines principles from statistics, computer science, and domain-specific knowledge to analyze and interpret complex data. The primary goal of Data Science is to uncover hidden patterns, generate valuable insights, and drive data-driven decision-making across various sectors. Data scientists use tools and techniques such as machine learning, data mining, and big data analytics to process large volumes of data and transform it into actionable information [10]. Today, Data Science is crucial for a wide range of applications, including business intelligence, healthcare analytics, financial forecasting, and personalized marketing, helping organizations enhance their operations and strategic planning.

A brief timeline of Data Science evolution covering past few decades has been illustrated in Fig. 2.12:

Starting in 1962, John Tukey's work on data analysis laid the groundwork for the field. The term "Data Science" was first used in 1974 by Peter Naur [11]. The introduction of the Box-Jenkins model in 1977 provided a comprehensive methodology for time series forecasting. The formalization of Knowledge Discovery in Databases (KDD) in 1989 and the rise of data warehousing in the 1990s further advanced the field. In 1995, the CRoss Industry Standard Process for Data Mining (CRISP-DM) methodology offered a structured approach to data mining projects. The early 2000s saw the recognition of data science as a discipline by William S. Cleveland and the launch of Apache Hadoop in 2005, revolutionizing data processing and storage.

The 2010s witnessed exponential growth in data science, driven by technological advancements and increased data availability. The introduction of Big Data in 2006, the emergence of the data scientist job title in 2009, and the development of Apache Spark in 2010 were pivotal. By 2012, data science was dubbed the "Sexiest Job of the 21st Century" by Harvard Business Review [12]. Python became the dominant programming language in 2014, enhancing data science's accessibility. The success of deep learning models in 2017, the release of Google's Bidirectional Encoder Representations from Transformers (BERT) for Natural Language Processing in 2018, and the convergence of AI and data science with OpenAI's GPT-3 in 2020 highlighted the field's progress. In 2023, the development of cloud-based platforms made advanced data analytics and machine learning more accessible, marking the latest milestone in the dynamic evolution of data science.

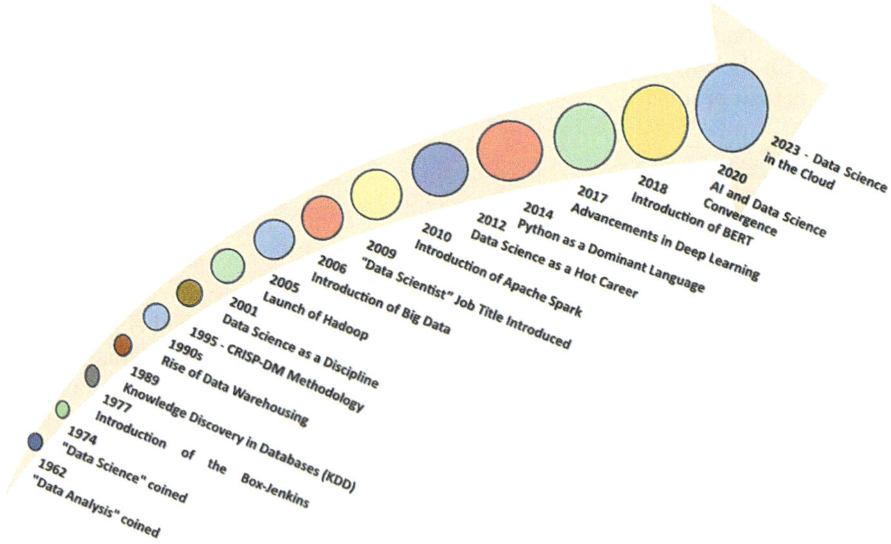

Fig. 2.12 Timeline for Data Science evolution

2.3.1 Key Techniques of DS

Firstly, statistical analysis, including descriptive statistics like mean, median, and standard deviation, and inferential statistics such as hypothesis testing, confidence intervals, and ANOVA, are used for interpreting data distributions and relationships. Deep learning techniques, particularly neural networks like CNNs, RNNs, and GANs, are employed for modeling complex patterns. Natural language processing (NLP) facilitates text mining, sentiment analysis, and machine translation, enhancing the interpretation of textual data. Time series analysis and forecasting, including trend analysis and seasonal decomposition, are crucial for predicting future data points. Pattern recognition through anomaly detection and signal processing identifies irregularities within data sets. Moreover, Big data analytics, leveraging data processing tools like Hadoop and Spark and storage solutions such as NoSQL databases and data warehousing, manages extensive datasets efficiently.

Data visualization, through interactive dashboards like Tableau and Power BI, and various graphical representations, simplifies data interpretation. Data mining techniques, including association rules, cluster analysis, and predictive modeling, uncover hidden patterns and trends. Optimization methods, including linear, integer, and non-linear programming, refine decision-making processes. Data engineering ensures seamless data flow through ETL processes, pipeline management, and integration into data lakes and warehouses. Finally, Artificial intelligence has been integrated with the DS tools, which is one of the recent breakthroughs in the domain. AI deploys knowledge representation, expert systems, planning and scheduling, and robotics, along with machine learning techniques such as supervised, unsupervised, and reinforcement learning, for reshaping data processing and analysis (Fig. 2.13).

2.3.2 Key Applications of DS

The core applications of Data Science span across various industries, driving innovation and enhancing efficiency. From healthcare and finance to retail and manufacturing, Data Science technologies are transforming how businesses operate and how services are delivered. By leveraging advanced analytics and data processing, Data Science enables informed decision-making, optimization, and personalized experiences, making it an indispensable tool in the modern world. Some of the major applications of Data Science have been listed in Fig. 2.14.

As previously discussed, the use of DS for healthcare combines data from multiple sources and provides a greater insight into the medical and disease history of the patient, improving the predictive analytics about the future health risks and disease progression. This is not only limited to individual patients, but also holds true for population health management. The advanced tools of DS, particularly Big Data Analytics algorithms facilitate quicker processing of massive real-time data collected from various sources; this benefit of DS is associated with accurate diagnosis,

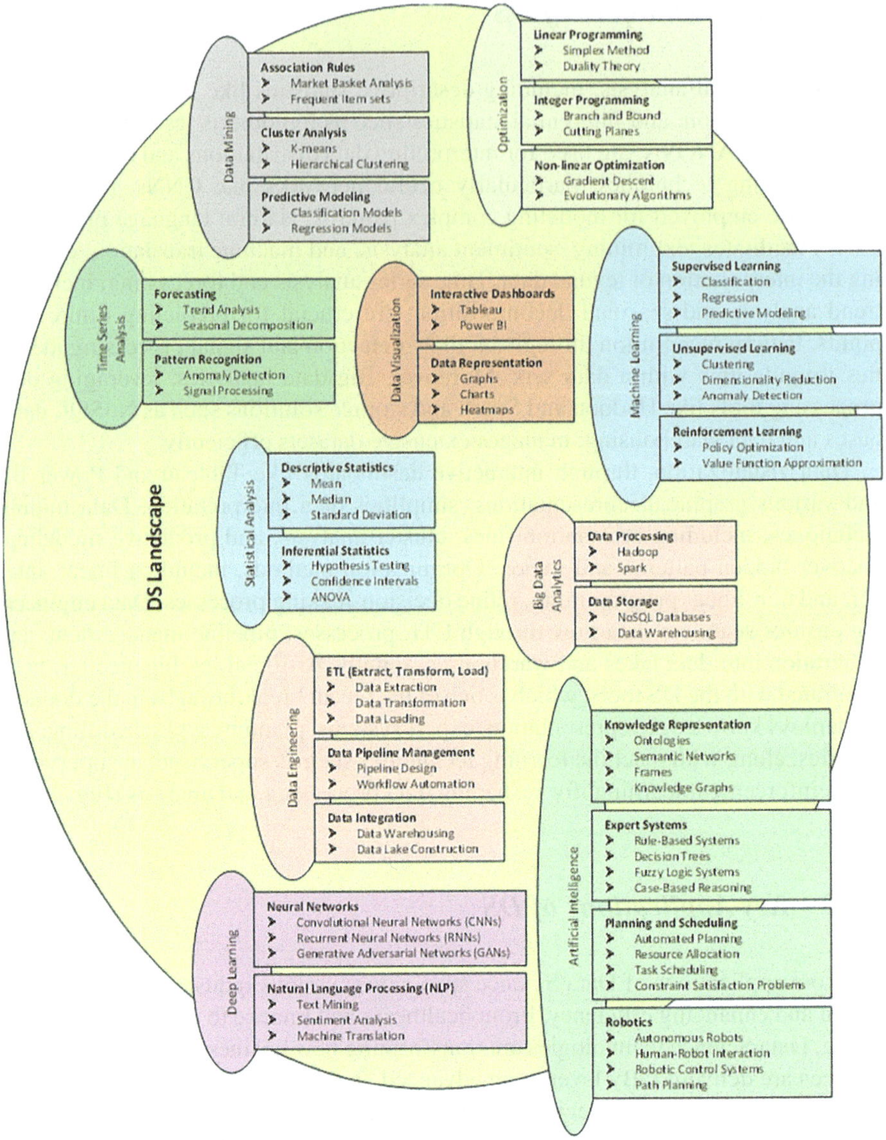

Fig. 2.13 DS techniques

pattern recognition and faster drug development. Clinical decision support systems are largely facilitated by Data science due to offering an insight into the large volumes of data in an organized and comprehensive manner, often using customized reports and visuals.

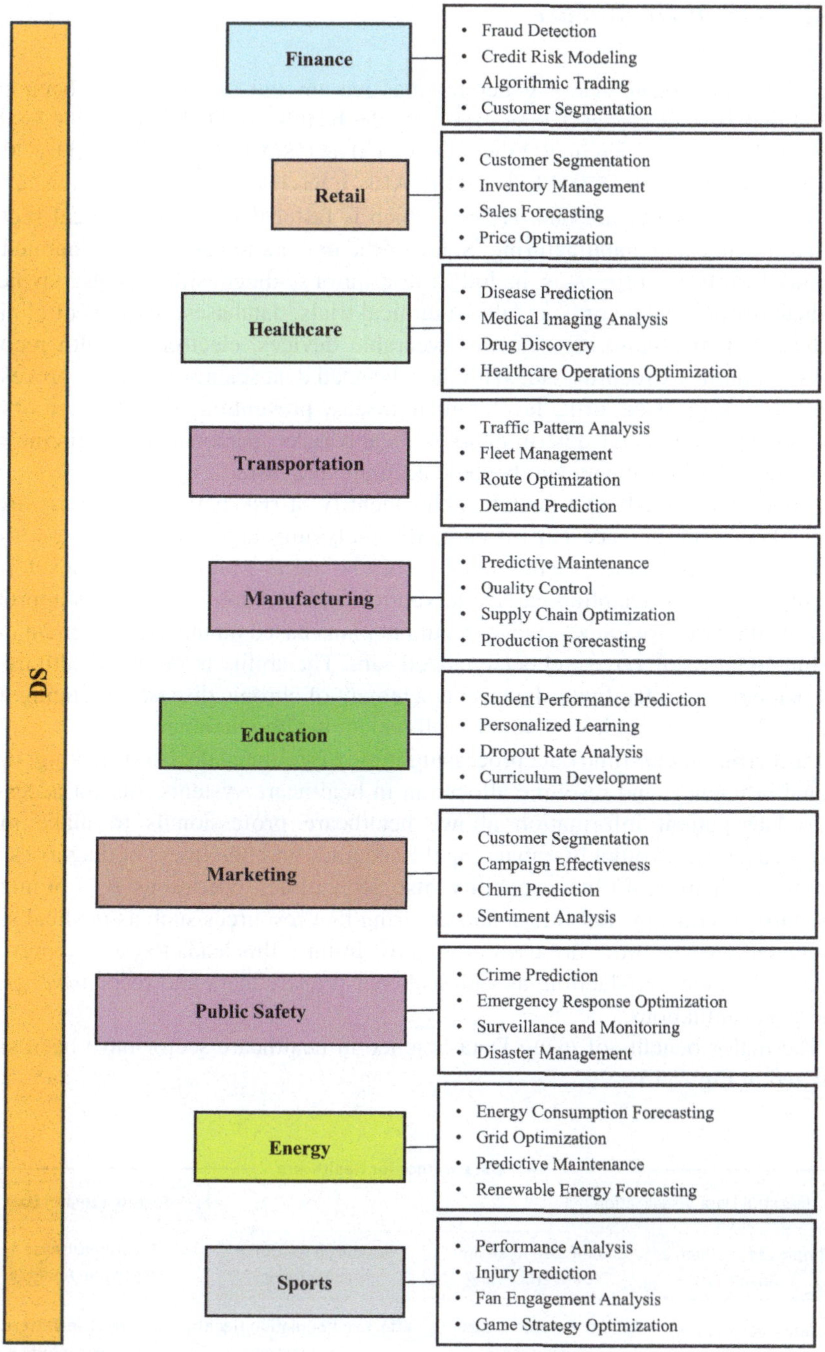

Fig. 2.14 Key applications of DS

2.3.3 DS in Healthcare

The global healthcare sector generates massive amount of data; it has been estimated that 30% of global data comes from the healthcare [13]. The global healthcare big data market size in 2023 was estimated as USD 42.64 billion, and by 2032, it is predicted to reach 137.05 billion [14]. Also, it has been estimated that the annual growth rate of healthcare data is 36% which is faster than several critical sectors such as finance and manufacturing. Some of the major sources of data generated by various healthcare processes include prescriptions, diagnostic reports, invoices, medical history and records, results of clinical trials, databases, findings of clinical studies, patient monitoring systems, wearable devices, electronic health records (EHRs), pharmacy records, etc. With the advanced data science tools, the processes of disease progression, drug development, disease prevention, identification of disease spread, and social determinants of health risks, personalized medicine and population health management become accurate and faster.

Additionally, predictive analytics can identify at-risk patients, optimize treatment plans, and enhance patient care. By analyzing large datasets from various sources, predictive models can flag patients who are at a higher risk of developing certain conditions, enabling early intervention and preventive care. This approach helps healthcare providers to tailor treatment plans based on individual patient data, leading to more effective and personalized care. The ability to predict health trends and outcomes also facilitates better management of chronic diseases, reducing hospital readmissions and improving overall patient health outcomes.

Furthermore, real-time data processing improves clinical decision-making, operational efficiency, and resource allocation in healthcare systems. Instant access to up-to-date patient information allows healthcare professionals to make more informed decisions quickly, enhancing the accuracy and timeliness of diagnoses and treatments. This real-time capability also streamlines operations by optimizing scheduling, reducing wait times, and ensuring that resources such as medical staff, equipment, and facilities are used efficiently. In turn, this leads to cost savings and improved patient satisfaction, as well as better preparedness and responsiveness in emergency situations.

The major benefits of using Data Science in healthcare sector have been summarized in Fig. 2.15:

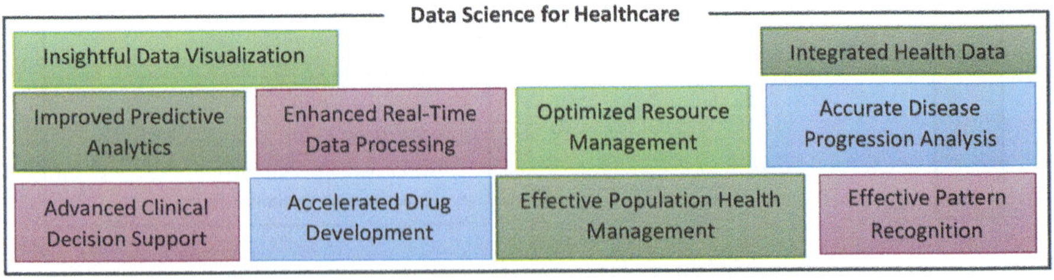

Fig. 2.15 Benefits of Data Science for healthcare

References

1. IoT connections worldwide 2022–2033 | Statista. Accessed 28 July 2024. [Online]. Available: https://www.statista.com/statistics/1183457/iot-connected-devices-worldwide/
2. R. Salama, C. Altrjman, F. Al-Turjman, An overview of the Internet of Things (IoT) and Machine to Machine (M2M) communications. NEU J. Artif. Intell. Internet Things **2**(3) (2023). Accessed 28 July 2024. [Online]. Available: https://dergi.neu.edu.tr/index.php/aiit/article/view/728
3. M. Lombardi, F. Pascale, D. Santaniello, Internet of things: A general overview between architectures, protocols and applications. Information **12**(2), 87 (2021). https://doi.org/10.3390/INFO12020087
4. I. Ghebrehiwet, N. Zaki, R. Damseh, M.S. Mohamad, Revolutionizing personalized medicine with generative AI: A systematic review. Artif. Intell. Rev. **57**(5), 1–41 (2024). https://doi.org/10.1007/S10462-024-10768-5/TABLES/6
5. P. Toupas, G. Tsamis, A. Kargakos, D. Giakoumis, K. Votis, D. Tzovaras, A framework towards ambient assisted living enhanced by service robots, in *ACM International Conference Proceeding Series*, (2023). https://doi.org/10.1145/3594806.3596532
6. R. Raj, A. Kos, Artificial intelligence: Evolution, developments, applications, and future scope. Prz. Elektrotech. **99**(2), 1 (2023). https://doi.org/10.15199/48.2023.02.01
7. A. Piorkowski, R. Obuchowicz, R. Najjar, Redefining radiology: A review of artificial intelligence integration in medical imaging. Diagnostics **13**(17), 2760 (2023). https://doi.org/10.3390/DIAGNOSTICS13172760
8. A.P. Zhao et al., AI for science: Predicting infectious diseases. J. Saf. Sci. Resil. **5**(2), 130–146 (2024). https://doi.org/10.1016/J.JNLSSR.2024.02.002
9. A. Blanco-González et al., The role of AI in drug discovery: Challenges, opportunities, and strategies. Pharmaceuticals **16**(6), 891 (2023). https://doi.org/10.3390/PH16060891/S1
10. A. Ahmed, R. Xi, M. Hou, S.A. Shah, S. Hameed, Harnessing big data analytics for healthcare: A comprehensive review of frameworks, implications, applications, and impacts. IEEE Access **11**, 112891–112928 (2023). https://doi.org/10.1109/ACCESS.2023.3323574
11. M.K.M. Nasution, R. Syah, M. Elveny, What is Data Science, in *Data Science with Semantic Technologies: New Trends and Future Developments*, (2023), pp. 1–25. https://doi.org/10.1201/9781003310785-1/DATA-SCIENCE-MAHYUDDIN-NASUTION-RAHMAD-SYAH-MARISCHA-ELVENY
12. E. Young, J. Wajcman, L. Sprejer, Mind the gender gap: Inequalities in the emergent professions of artificial intelligence (AI) and data science. N. Technol. Work. Employ. **38**(3), 391–414 (2023). https://doi.org/10.1111/NTWE.12278
13. How healthcare data technology is leveraged by leaders. Accessed 29 July 2024. [Online]. Available: https://arcadia.io/resources/healthcare-data-technology
14. Global Big Data in healthcare market size, top share, trends, report to 2032. Accessed 29 July 2024. [Online]. Available: https://straitsresearch.com/report/big-data-in-healthcare-market

Chapter 3
Innovations in Continuous Patient Monitoring

3.1 Foundations of Continuous Monitoring

Conventionally, the continuous monitoring, specifically, remote was meant for the patients belonging from the rural areas or those who suffer from the chronic diseases. However, since the COVID period, the continuous monitoring of hospitalized patients has also become a norm; this not only ensures better quality of care for the patients but also reduces burden on the hospitals due to the reduction in staff visits to each patient. Mostly, the starting point of the continuous monitoring technology is either wearable or ambient sensor. The network formed by wearable devices is often termed as Wireless Body Area Network (WBAN), and when it connects to the personal handheld devices and computers, it is enhanced to Personal Area Network (PAN).

Initially, the focus of wearable devices was only on real-time communication about patients' state to the remote caregivers, which was mainly served by IoT or IoMT (Internet of Medical Things). However, as the technology evolved, advanced techniques from the domains of DS and AI also began to be applied on the continuous data streams received from the patients. The role of each technology in the IoT-DS-AI nexus has been illustrated in Fig. 3.1:

3.2 IoT: The Data Collecting Technology

As earlier illustrated in Fig. 2.2, the basic architecture of IoT involves collecting data from sensors, processing it over handheld device (edge computing) and forward it to fog or cloud layer. This section describes the key protocols used for IoT communication, the features of underlying software (the mobile apps) and the cloud platform.

S. Siddiqui et al., *Connected Health Insights for Sustainable Development*,
https://doi.org/10.1007/978-3-031-81433-4_3

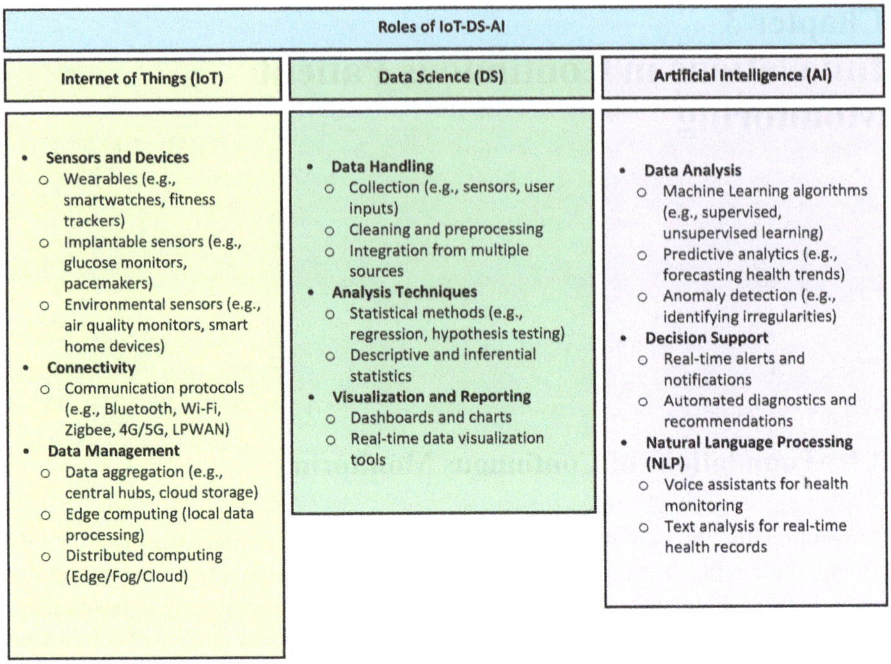

Fig. 3.1 Role of IoT, DS and AI for continuous monitoring application

3.2.1 Sensors

Various sensors are used for continuous patient monitoring, with the choice largely governed by the application. For example, heart rate monitors use optical sensors to detect blood flow, while accelerometers and gyroscopes measure movement and posture. Temperature sensors track body heat, and electrocardiogram (ECG) sensors monitor heart rhythms. Additionally, glucose sensors are employed for diabetes management, and pulse oximeters measure oxygen saturation levels. Most of these sensors are embedded within the wearable devices such as smart watches or wristbands; however, there are also commercial variant of the conventional vital measuring devices that embed Bluetooth modules. With the help of Bluetooth enabled devices such as blood pressure or Glucose monitors, there is a significant enhancement in the scope of continuous monitoring applications; use of communication protocols within the conventional medical devices helps to reduce the digital divide; for example, the elderly or majority users from under-developed regions might not be able to use even the simplest of health monitoring mobile apps, however, they can comfortably use the Bluetooth-enabled medical devices, which would directly input the measured values into the relevant mobile app, for subsequent transmission to the central dashboards and physicians' app interfaces. Today, we even have ingestible and implantable sensors that track the parameters which are not possible to be collected from on-body devices. These sensors can be thought of as an advanced version of pacemakers as they can also transmit data using advanced means of wireless communication such as molecular and THz [1].

In addition to the wearable sensors or connected medical devices, ambient sensors are also used for continuous monitoring. The concept of AAL has already been discussed in Sect. 2.1.3; the AAL has been derived from the two areas of "Ambient intelligence" and "Assisted Living", and makes use of emerging computing and communication technologies for facilitating the independently living elderly. The drivers for the recent increase in the acceptance of AAL technology is the globally increasing elderly population, known deterioration of their physical and mental health and the long hours they spend at home, usually alone.

The goal of AAL technology is to detect the presence of users, recognize their activities, detect behaviors and report to the interested stakeholders [2]. In this context, various sensors are used such as light, temperature, humidity, vibration, sound, air quality, of course, camera. These ambient sensors enhance the capability to monitor and analyze the environment, providing comprehensive data that can be used to improve patient care, detect anomalies, optimize energy consumption, and ensure safety. Novel applications of AAL integrating IoT, AI and DS have been proposed; for example, an alert could be generated for the family members in case an elderly patient does not get out of bed by a certain time; this information can be detected by applying ML and DL algorithms received from camera feed. Similarly, the use of bathroom showers or kitchen coffee makers can provide an insight into the health states of patients. By integrating data from various sources, it is possible to gain a holistic understanding of the patient's environment and health status, leading to more accurate and timely interventions.

3.2.2 Key Protocols

Recently, various short-range protocols are being developed for IoT devices such as WiFi, Zigbee, BLE and Bluetooth. The choice of protocol is dependent on the bandwidth requirement which is application-specific; for example, BLE could easily be used for a sensor signal that requires 0.5 Hz, such as SPO_2 signal. On the other hand, if the application is set to send 25 lead ECG signals with a bandwidth requirement of 500 Hz, WiFi should be used for meeting the required quality. Some of the key IoT protocols used in healthcare are illustrated in Fig. 3.2, in terms of their range and data rate.

Many of the recent protocols shown in Fig. 3.2 are designed with the features of low cost, low energy consumption and low bit rate, while operating over Low Power Wide-Area Networks (LPWAN). Some examples include NB-IoT, Sigfox and LoRaWAN. Another common feature of these protocols is their capability to connect a large number of devices. To exemplify these features, we may consider IEEE 802.15.6 standard, that supports data rates up to 10 Mbps within a range of 1–2 m, while ensuring low power consumption and high reliability [3]. Recent advancements in IoT communication infrastructure feature the latest 3GPP standards

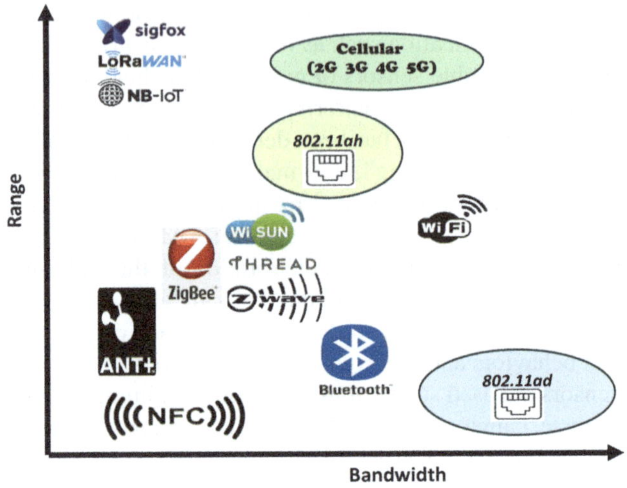

Fig. 3.2 Comparing Recent Protocols of IoT in terms of Range and Bandwidth

development for 5G IoT, aimed at providing low-power, low-data-rate, and wide-area coverage for various IoT devices. This development includes two types of connections: direct 3GPP connection via narrowband IoT (NB-IoT) and indirect non-3GPP connection. NB-IoT requires only 180 kHz of bandwidth for both uplink and downlink. To support non-3GPP 5G IoT connections, combining a low-power wide-area network (LPWAN) with cellular networks through relay user equipment (UE) offers a promising solution.

3.2.3 Mobile Applications

Various mobile apps have been developed to provide an interface between the devices and users. The apps are commonly used for remote health monitoring for offering device to device communication (often termed as Machine-to-Machine or M2M communication), device to human and human to human communication [3]. Based on the patient requirement, the app should be accessible, present information in an intuitive manner, present the solutions to patients' problems, and collect their feedback. Particularly for the remote and continuous health monitoring purposes, the app should seamlessly connect with the wearable devices [4]. Mostly the health apps are used by fitness enthusiasts or chronic patients. Some of the major features healthcare apps should offer are listed below:

Measurement: It often involves device-to-device communication; for example, for monitoring blood pressure or blood sugar, the relevant devices of glucometers or sphygmomanometer generally communicate with the hand-held devices. The users may see their statistics and attempt modifying their lifestyle/diet and habits to improve the trends.

Maintaining History: This is related to device-to-human interaction. The patients as well as physicians can see the health trends as and when required. This is an essential feature of continuous health monitoring apps as it reduces the burden of managing health records and offers a detailed insight not only into the health trends, but also into the previous diagnostics, prescriptions, etc.

Survey Questionnaires: In addition to the wearable or other medical equipment connecting to the hand-held devices, it is also a norm to ask users about their health/wellness. These questionnaires are commonly used for chronic and mental health issues. This feature exemplifies device-to-human communication.

Training and Awareness: This feature also belongs from the category of device-to-human communication. The users are often offered health training and awareness using their mobile phone. These are low-cost and effective awareness programs, due to their customization for specific patients, designed based on their health stats. Today, advanced AI tools have been such as generative AI have been used for providing customized services such as therapies, diagnosis, etc. [4].

Diary and Reminders: A common feature offered by mobile apps is to provide reminders to the patients about their upcoming appointments, medicines, exercise and diet routines etc. This helps patients stay organized and adhere to their treatment plans more effectively. This functionality represents a crucial aspect of device-to-human interaction, where technology is utilized to support and enhance patient engagement and self-management of their health. Moreover, mobile apps can send real-time alerts and notifications for critical health events. For example, if a patient's heart rate exceeds a certain threshold, the app can immediately notify the patient and their healthcare provider. This feature ensures timely medical intervention, which is the most critical requirement of continuous monitoring.

Communication and Collaboration: The modern apps also provide multi-user and community interfaces for human-to-human communication. Using this feature, the patients may talk to their physicians, to their family members or extended community; in fact, today, healthcare apps also provide an opportunity to physicians for sharing medical advice or patient history. This concept has already been discussed in Sect. 2.1.3.

Emergency Response: Certain apps are equipped with emergency response features, which could trigger certain pre-defined actions in case of vitals reaching a threshold, or patients' actions such as use of a panic button. Such actions may alert emergency contacts and provide the user's location in case of a medical emergency. Moreover, the emergency service providers such as ambulance services can also be timely intimidated. This feature adds an extra layer of security for patients with serious health conditions. It can be categorized as device-to-human and/or human-to-human interaction.

Further details on health-specific mobile applications are discussed in Chap. 5.

3.2.4 Cloud Computing

Cloud services are used for continuous health monitoring in order to perform various tasks on the data obtained from different wearable/ambient sensors and devices. First and foremost, these platforms provide infrastructure to store and organize the data; these also provide servers for processing the collected data, intelligent systems for producing alerts and assist physicians in the decision-making. By considering a specific patient example, we may clarify the role of each component: the server is responsible for storing the patient's vital data, the intelligent (feature extraction) module analyses the patient data and extract high-level features/trends from the raw patient data, and finally, the decision support system (DSS) uses dynamic rules to assess the physicians in their clinical decision making.

Deploying cloud into the IoT architecture ensures that the patient data will remain protected and available whenever needed. In this context, various cloud architectures including Infrastructure as a Service (IaaS), Platform as a service (PaaS) or Software as a Service (SaaS) are available to be used for healthcare applications. The cloud platforms commonly used for the continuous health monitoring, along with their characteristics have been summarized Fig. 3.3:

In addition to the features shown above, the selection criteria for cloud services also include pricing model, flexibility and deployment type. Flexibility, scalability and interoperability are the core design features of cloud services and these are essential for the remote health monitoring applications. Hence, to achieve interoperability, HL7 FHIR is adopted which is an electronic health record handling standard and ensures seamless integration between heterogenous systems. Moreover, flexibility and scalability are addressed through ensuring that the cloud APIs would not need to be changed while adding the new resources to the network.

3.3 DS: The Data Processing Technology

Once the data is collected by the wearable and sent to the hand-held device, and subsequently to the cloud, the role of DS comes into play. Various techniques of data science starting at mere data aggregation and extending to complex big data analytics techniques are applied to achieve the desired goals of risk identification for the patients being continuously monitored. Once the data is cleaned and pre-processed, analytics and visualization are the major DS techniques that add value to the continuous monitoring applications. This section addresses the major DS techniques involved including time series analysis, predictive analytics, clustering, anomaly detection and data visualization.

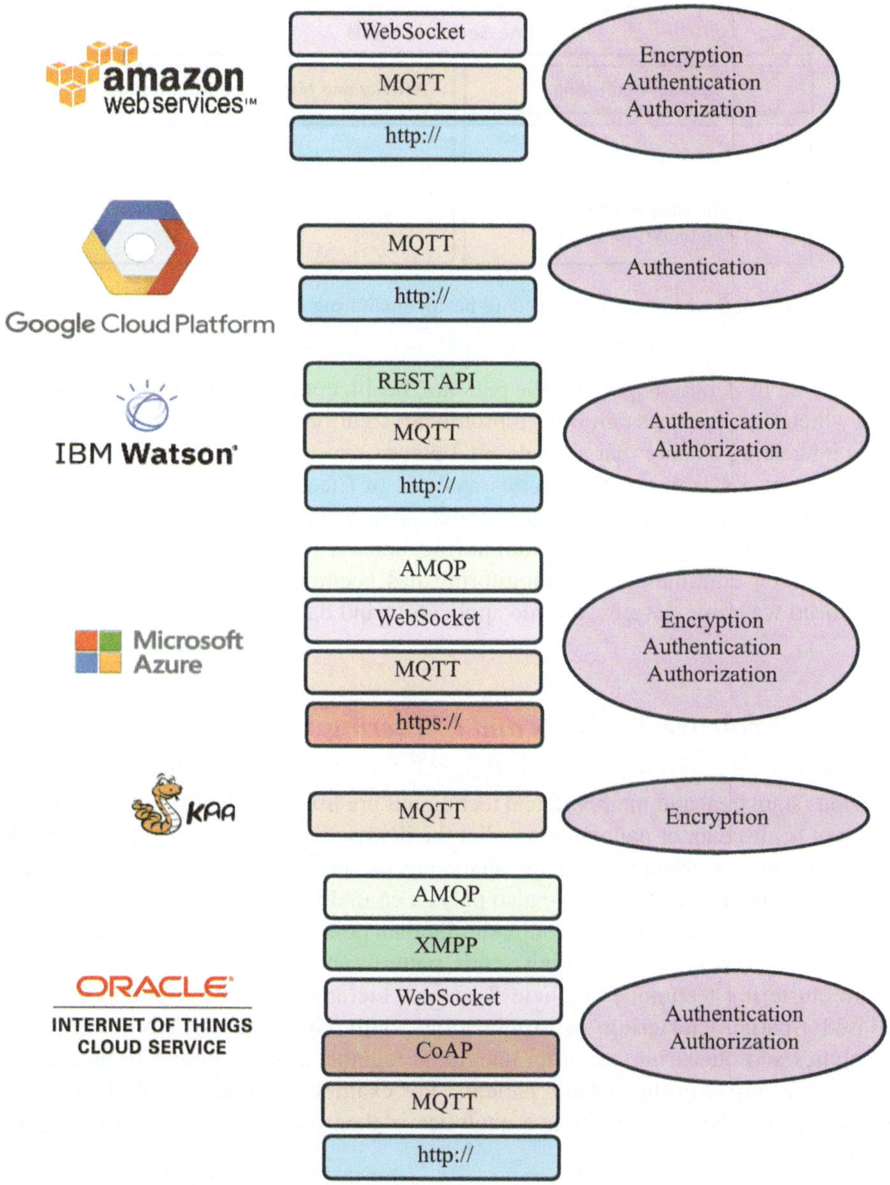

Fig. 3.3 Cloud platforms and their features

3.3.1 Time Series Analysis

Timer series analysis can easily be integrated with continuous/remote patient monitoring applications, as most of the scenarios are designed to collect and report continuous vital data. Particularly for chronic patients, the time series analysis would

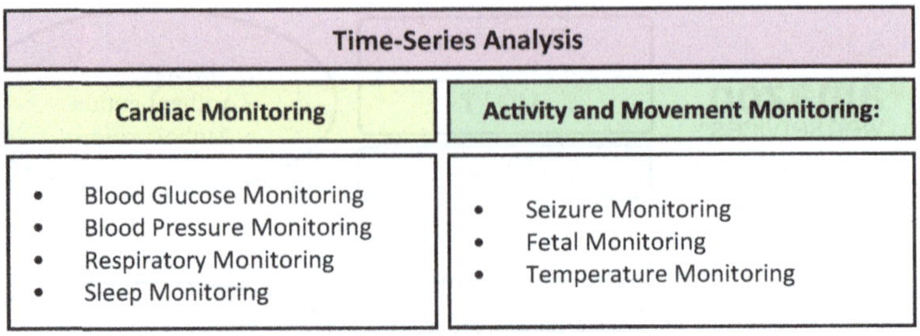

Fig. 3.4 Time series analysis for continuous health monitoring

provide an in-depth insight into the patients' health condition. Some of the diseases for which time analysis can offer a promising solution are summarized in Fig. 3.4. It is interesting to note that a single vital parameter can be used for more than one application; for example, time-series analysis of Electrocardiogram (ECG) would not only provide general information about the heart health, but can also be used for the applications of sleep quality monitoring, activity monitoring and seizure monitoring. Even continuous fetal monitoring has become possible with the help of advanced wearable devices, mobile application and data analytics [5].

3.3.2 Predictive Analytics and Clustering

Various statistical and mathematical techniques are used for identifying the past and present health data of patients to predict the disease risk. Regression analysis is the most common technique used for analyzing the patterns of vital parameters and detect the risk levels. Clustering also plays a crucial role for the continuous patient monitoring applications as it groups similar data points (similar values of vital signs in our case). It helps in identifying trends, patterns and anomalies. Some of the common clustering techniques include K-means, hierarchical clustering and Density-Based Spatial Clustering of Applications with Noise (DBSCAN). Predictive analytics and clustering are often integrated together when it comes to predict the patterns of vitals in the chronic patients. For example, similar values of vitals are clustered together, and predictive analytics is then used for predicting the future situation.

3.3.3 Anomaly Detection

Anomaly detection holds importance for the continuous monitoring patient as it may deviate the entire trend of monitored data, if not efficiently dealt with. If anomalies are not properly addressed, they could result in misinterpretation of diagnosis;

for example, if the blood pressure or blood sugar value shows a certain spike, it could be just an anomaly, but it could also be a critical event for the patient. Also, the patients could also unknowingly be responsible for recording outlier values, in case they do not observe the necessary precautions given by the app or doctor. As an example, we may consider a chronic hypertension patient who is using a continuous monitoring mobile health app; this patient uses a Bluetooth enabled sphygmomanometer to periodically record their blood pressure via mobile app. The patient has been advised not to measure the values after 30 min of exercise; now, in case the patient is showing a stable trend otherwise, but just one time, they do not take care of the waiting precaution after exercise, there will be a clear disruption in the entire trend. Same situations may also happen due to technical malfunction of the devices or connectivity issues, where certain values might not be uploaded to the cloud, although correctly measured by the devices. Hence, it becomes crucial to detect and delete the outlier values.

Some of the major statistical techniques of anomaly detection include Z-score, Grubb's test and Chi-Square test. Z-Score measures how many standard deviations a data point is from the mean. A high Z-score indicates a potential anomaly. **Grubbs' Test** identifies outliers in a univariate dataset using statistical tests and by assuming that the data is normally distributed. Finally, **Chi-Square Test** is used for categorical data to detect anomalies by comparing observed frequencies with expected frequencies. For the continuous monitoring application, Z-score is more likely to be used as it suits more for the real-time continuous data streams; it would help to detect unusual patient metrics like blood pressure, glucose levels, or heart rate. Moreover, this score is also easy and quick to calculate and interpret which is one of the core requirements of remote health monitoring systems as it is crucial to reach quickly to the inference, for subsequent intervention planning.

3.3.4 Data Visualization

For visualizing the patients' data on central dashboards or hand-held devices, DS offers various reporting tools. The global healthcare data analytics industry is expected to grow up to $85.9 billion in 2027 [6]. Customized dashboards and graphs are developed for providing a quick overview of patient's health to the physicians. The visualization tools offer various benefits including improved patient care, trends and pattern recognition, as well as detection of errors/frauds. The modern tools can offer user-friendly and interactive interfaces for presenting the complex data, and their associations. For example, instead of looking at long logs of medical history, a physician or caregiver is likely to be more interested in quickly looking at a graph that shows trend of patient's blood pressure over past 24 h. The most common choices of medical visualization tools are discussed next.

3.3.5 *Interactive Dashboards*

Dashboards integrate data received from various sources and are known as one of the most common visualization tools. They are often built with data analysis functionalities, and even have ML components embedded. It is crucial to have efficient, fast and customized dashboards to facilitate the continuous patient monitoring functionality. There are three major types of dashboards: operational, strategic and analytical. The operational dashboard is used for displaying real-time patient data coming as a continuous stream; strategic dashboard is used for presenting the trends and patterns developed over time, and analytical dashboard provides more advanced tools for performing customized analytics.

3.3.6 *Interactive Apps and Sites*

Interactive apps and websites help the patients as well as physicians to quickly identify the important trends and other information. For example, based on the patient's vitals and emergency/risk level, their mobile health app may inform about the nearest available care provider. Similarly, the physicians might identify the patients with highest risk levels on their phone apps.

3.3.7 *Visualization Tools in Practice*

Commonly used visualization tools for the healthcare sector include Tableau and Power BI. Tableau is the most widely used due to its ability of handling large datasets. It also offers highly interactive and customized visualization while providing powerful data integration. Moreover, Microsoft's tool Power BI integrates well with other Microsoft products and offers robust data visualization and business intelligence capabilities.

3.4 AI: The Decision-Making Technology

AI has been used for data collected through IoT, and processed through DS while doing continuous patient monitoring. The major focus of this technology is on analyzing medical data and images while also corelating the clinical data such as biomarkers and symptoms; using all these information pieces, AI identifies the illnesses, as well as their prognosis. The advancement in the computation speed also contributes to more efficient real-time decision making while analyzing the complex patterns in the data received from patients. For example, Artificial Neural Networks and Deep Learning algorithms can now handle and optimize complex datasets quickly, assisting continuous monitoring; this was clearly not possible few years back. Commonly, AI methods are adopted for predicting vital signs and classifying the diseases or risk levels for patients being continuously monitored. Some of the major areas in which AI is being integrated with continuous monitoring applications are detailed below:

3.4.1 Monitoring Vital Signs

Wearable devices such as smart watches continuously track pulse rate and other vital parameters. Such devices generate bulk of data which can easily be used as input by key AI algorithms like Support Vector Machine (SVM). For example, the cloud server may use SVM for analysis of the continuous data stream, and the insights can be shared with patients as well as physicians. There is a high probability of diseases risk detection by these systems, which subsequently facilitate planning early interventions [5]. One such study was conducted in 2020 where decision tree classifier was trained for identifying ECG signals; 20-fold cross-validation and 31 features were used in the training of CatBoost learning kit. The topmost features were extracted based on their importance. The trained CatBoost model was able to process 30 s ECG data in 0.5 s, with an accuracy of 99.62% and sensitivity of 96.1% [7] Another study deployed IoT-based wearable 12-lead ECG SmartVest system for assessing ECG quality using SVM; the average accuracy achieved from this system was 97.9% and 96.4% for acceptable and unacceptable ECG segments, respectively [8] Similarly, there are various other examples where AI methods of Multilayer perceptron (MLP) neural network, recurrent neural network (RNN), deep convolutional neural network (DCNN), auto-encoder, restricted Boltzmann machine (RBM), and deep learning LSTM have been used for detecting cardiac diseases.

3.4.2 Monitoring Physical Activity

Powerful AI methods are also being used for activity recognition of the patients at risk. For example, a fall detection method has been developed using random forest (RF) algorithm that works by fusing data collected through various sensors as well as camera (feature). The researchers have even conducted simulation studies where hundreds of volunteers have participated for making the algorithms learn the activities and fall movements. Similarly, multiphase falls identification algorithms have been developed using ML techniques, where the goal is not only to detect fall, but also the stages of pre-fall, free-fall, impact, resting. These algorithms make use of more than one ML technique including SVM, KNN, naive Bayes, decision tree, and adaptive boosting [9]. Moreover, signal reflection model has also been used for detecting fall, where the strength of RSSI from RFID tag is monitored. Again, various ML classifiers are used for the purpose including RF, multilayer Perceptron-based Neural Network, Decision Tree, SVM, Naive Bayes, and Quadratic Discriminant Analysis [10]; this approach also identifies various activities such as raising the hand up or down, walking, sitting, falling, rotating and no activity.

3.4.3 Monitoring Chronic Diseases

As mentioned earlier, managing chronic illnesses remains one of the major causes of using technology for continuous monitoring. AI has widely been used for modeling the risks and predicting the occurrences of issues such as cardiac diseases, diabetes, pain and chronic respiratory conditions. AI and ML algorithms can be deployed for analyzing large amounts of patient data in real-time, to identify patterns and potential health risks; this proactive approach helps them to plan early interventions before the risks become critical and life-threatening. In this context, various studies have been done for predicting diabetes. For example, external factors other than blood Glucose Levels could also be considered for modeling the diabetes risk as done in [11], where ML algorithms SVM, Decision Tree, Extra Tree, Neural Networks, Ada Boost, Gaussian Naïve Bayes, K-Nearest Neighbor, Logistic Regression and Gradient Boost Classifier have been used. The external factors evaluated in this study included age, insulin dosage and Body Mass Index (BMI). Similarly, AI can also be used for innovative applications for diabetic patients; for example, ANN and SVM have been used for predicting the best exercise routines based on the blood sugar levels [12]. AI can also be used for pain management through continuous monitoring; the wearable device and mobile apps are integrated together to record the pain levels and identify the pain patterns. As a result of this analysis, developing customized pain management strategies becomes possible.

Several commercial solutions have also been made available that help to track the vital signs and detect disease risks using AI. For Example, AliveCor provides AI-driven ECG monitors that patients can use at home; the product uses AI algorithms to analyze ECG to detect abnormalities such as atrial fibrillation, arrhythmias, and other cardiac conditions [13]. Similarly, IBM Watson Health uses AI to identify patients at risk of heart failure [14]; the company's solutions in addition to monitoring vitals, also monitor the lifestyle factors such as diet and fitness routines, genetic information and medical history to predict the likelihood of heart attacks or strokes. AI tools have also been used form monitoring chronic respiratory conditions; Propeller Health's smart inhalers track medication usage and environmental factors to predict and prevent asthma attacks or COPD exacerbations [15]. Moreover, AI algorithms are also capable to assess spirometry data to assess lung function and predict the progression of respiratory diseases.

In addition to above, there are several innovative and unconventional AI models trained for continuous monitoring solutions. Google AI subsidiary DeepMind developed an ML model for predicting kidney injuries [16]. The team did a study on a large dataset and the model was able to predict kidney injury up to 48 h in advance. Clearly, this time margin would allow the physicians to intervene and treat the patient, saving them from life-threatening situations. As another disruption to the conventional diagnostics, Food and Drug Administration (FDA) has approved several AI tools for screening cancers of brain, breast, lung, prostate, skin, and thyroid [17]. The major reason behind success of AI for predicting the cancer is its ability of analyze image based on its training that is done on million of images. Such accurate and vast knowledge is never possible to be contained within a human brain, hence, AI surpasses human decision making for cancer detection.

3.5 Mental Health Monitoring

Mental health has also been facilitated by AI for predicting various conditions such as bipolar disorder, suicidal tendency, major depressive disorder and schizophrenia. Initially, various mobile apps were developed for identifying the issues such as anxiety and depressions only to facilitate the remote consultation and counseling. Subsequently, trend monitoring was included in the apps so the patients and physicians can have an insight into the occurrence of anxiety/depression episodes. Today, we have advanced AI algorithms embedded with the mental health mobile apps and digital platforms. These algorithms identify the symptoms and risk factors for mental health issues. Moreover, AI techniques also help to predict the progression of disease, which is then used for developing customized therapies and other treatment strategies. Recently, the concept of Conversational AI agents has also been proposed where chatbots play the role of psychologists and develop a human-AI therapeutic relationships [18]. Such techniques of using AI for offering therapy and counseling would not only make the mental healthcare more effective, but will also make the service more accessible by eliminating the taboo associated with receiving therapy in a conventional setting.

The use of AI for mental health has particularly been affected by the recent development of Chat Generative Pre-training Transformer (ChatGPT), which is a powerful AI-based chatbot. The bot utilizes transformer-based neural network system, that makes it capable of producing human-like content [19]. ChatGPT has the capability of responding to the users in a conversation style as it is trained on Large Language Model (LLM). Due to the diverse capabilities of ChatGPT such as writing papers, composing music, writing computer programs, offering counseling etc.; therefore, the tool is expected to impact the mental healthcare delivery positively by offering free services any time. With the development of ChatGPT, the users would not even need to have access to any dedicated mobile app; rather they can just log in at any time and can ask questions from the bot. For example, if a mother is feeling anxiety due to postpartum depression, she can seek help from ChatGPT and same is valid for the elderly who might need an assistant just for chatting. Since ChatGPT is a multilingual platform, this feature would also add to the flexibility it could offer to the users.

3.6 Continuous Patient Monitoring Leading to SDG 3

The use of IoT, AI and DS for continuous patient monitoring at home or hospitals has a considerable potential for contributing towards achieving SDG 3. First and foremost, these technologies provide access to healthcare for those who live at remote areas, for those who could not afford to visit expert clinics, and also for those who avoid to avail care due to social taboos (such as women not receiving reproductive care or people in general not receiving psychological counseling). Secondly, chronic disease monitoring and management becomes very cost-effective and easy using the technology, which is not possible otherwise. People suffering from chronic diseases (majority elderly) often tend to miss their medicine and doctor's appointments due to forgetfulness or busy schedules. With the help of continuous monitoring, their health state is always communicated to the doctors, regardless of whether the patients show up on the scheduled appointment. As a matter of fact, the continuous monitoring facilities even outperform the conventional check ups method because following that, the patients interact with the doctors only once in a while, whereas while using wearable and other technologies discusses in the chapter, the patients always remain connected. There are various proposals in literature and some commercial implementations where the doctors can find the risk levels of each patient for various diseases on central dashboards [20].

Hence, the technologies presented in this chapter can ensure healthy lives and promote well-being for all regardless of their location, age and economic class.

References

1. K. Yang et al., A comprehensive survey on hybrid communication in context of molecular communication and terahertz communication for body-centric nanonetworks. IEEE Trans. Mol. Biol. Multiscale Commun. **6**(2) (2020). https://doi.org/10.1109/TMBMC.2020.3017146
2. E. Sulis et al., An ambient assisted living architecture for hospital at home coupled with a process-oriented perspective. J. Ambient. Intell. Humaniz. Comput. **15**(5) (2024). https://doi.org/10.1007/s12652-022-04388-6
3. N.Y. Philip, J.J.P.C. Rodrigues, H. Wang, S.J. Fong, J. Chen, Internet of things for in-home health monitoring systems: Current advances, challenges and future directions. IEEE J Sel Areas Commun **39**(2), 300–310 (2021). https://doi.org/10.1109/JSAC.2020.3042421
4. S. Saleh, B. Cherradi, O. El Gannour, N. Gouiza, O. Bouattane, Healthcare monitoring system for automatic database management using mobile application in IoT environment. Bull. Electr. Eng. Inform. **12**(2), 1055–1068 (2023). https://doi.org/10.11591/EEI.V12I2.4282
5. K.K. Tamber, D.J.L. Hayes, S.J. Carey, J.H.B. Wijekoon, A.E.P. Heazell, A systematic scoping review to identify the design and assess the performance of devices for antenatal continuous fetal monitoring. PLoS One **15**(12) (2020). https://doi.org/10.1371/journal.pone.0242983
6. Healthcare analytics market worth $85.9 billion by 2027. Accessed 03 Aug 2024. [Online]. Available: https://www.marketsandmarkets.com/PressReleases/healthcare-data-analytics.asp
7. B. Dhananjay, J. Sivaraman, Analysis and classification of heart rate using CatBoost feature ranking model. Biomed Signal. Process Control **68** (2021). https://doi.org/10.1016/j.bspc.2021.102610

8. M. Moshawrab, M. Adda, A. Bouzouane, H. Ibrahim, A. Raad, Smart wearables for the detection of cardiovascular diseases: A systematic literature review. Sensors (Basel) **23**(2), 828 (2023). https://doi.org/10.3390/s23020828
9. N. Thakur, C.Y. Han, A study of fall detection in assisted living: Identifying and improving the optimal machine learning method. J. Sens. Actuator Netw. **10**(3) (2021). https://doi.org/10.3390/jsan10030039
10. M.G.E. Ante, R. Gustilo, A.S.I. Crisostomo, S. Al Balushi, Human activity recognition using supervised machine learning techniques, in *AIP Conference Proceedings*, (2024). https://doi.org/10.1063/5.0194457
11. S.S. Bhat, M. Banu, G.A. Ansari, V. Selvam, A risk assessment and prediction framework for diabetes mellitus using machine learning algorithms. Healthc. Anal. **4**, 100273 (2023). https://doi.org/10.1016/j.health.2023.100273
12. A.A. Khan, S. Siddiqui, S.M. Shah, F. Nait-Abdesselam, I. Dey, Comparing ANN and SVM algorithms for predicting exercise routines of diabetic patients, in *2021 International Wireless Communications and Mobile Computing, IWCMC 2021*, (2021). https://doi.org/10.1109/IWCMC51323.2021.9498950
13. Alivecor | Alivecor Home. Accessed 03 Aug 2024. [Online]. Available: https://alivecor.com/
14. AI hot in healthcare despite IBM's Watson health pullout. Accessed 03 Aug 2024. [Online]. Available: https://www.labiotech.eu/trends-news/ibm-watson-health-ai/
15. Propeller Health: A Precision Digital Health Company. Accessed 03 Aug 2024. [Online]. Available: https://propellerhealth.com/
16. X. Yu, Y. Ji, M. Huang, Z. Feng, Machine learning for acute kidney injury: Changing the traditional disease prediction mode. Front. Med. **10**, 1050255 (2023). https://doi.org/10.3389/fmed.2023.1050255
17. Is it cancer? Artificial intelligence helps doctors get a clearer picture | AAMC. Accessed 03 Aug 2024. [Online]. Available: https://www.aamc.org/news/it-cancer-artificial-intelligence-helps-doctors-get-clearer-picture
18. H. Li, R. Zhang, Y.C. Lee, R.E. Kraut, D.C. Mohr, Systematic review and meta-analysis of AI-based conversational agents for promoting mental health and well-being. NPJ Digit. Med. **6**, 236 (2023). https://doi.org/10.1038/s41746-023-00979-5
19. O. Singh, Artificial intelligence in the era of ChatGPT-Opportunities and challenges in mental health care. Indian J. Psychiatry **65**(3), 297–298 (2023). https://doi.org/10.4103/indianjpsychiatry.indianjpsychiatry_112_23
20. S. Siddiqui, F. Nait-Abdesselam, A.A. Khan, I. Dey, Enabling real-time dashboards for anxiety risk classification using the internet of things, in *Proceedings—IEEE Global Communications Conference*, (GLOBECOM, 2021). https://doi.org/10.1109/GLOBECOM46510.2021.9685683

Chapter 4
Mobile Health (m-Health)

4.1 Defining m-Health

According to World Health Organization (WHO), Mobile Health (m-health) is defined as "the use of mobile wireless technologies for public health" [1]. Today, tens of healthcare mobile applications have been commercialized that either take input from wearable sensors, or from sensors embedded within the smart phones. These mobile apps help the patients to access continuous care at an affordable price, regardless of their physical location. The patients are empowered via m-Health for self-management of their health as they get customized tools to track various health metrics such as physical activity, diet, medication adherence, and vital signs. The quality and coverage of care significantly improves with the advent of m-health as compared to the conventional healthcare systems due to the increase in access to health services, skills and information. Moreover, the technology also promotes awareness and positive changes in lifestyle of users, which in turn, improves the chronic disease management probability. Let's look at the brief history and evolution of m-Health Concepts.

4.2 History and Evolution

The areas of mobile app development, wireless communications, IoT and AI have been increasingly integrated with healthcare. A brief timeline for m-health evolution has been illustrated in Fig. 4.1.

It was during 1980s that the concepts of telemedicine were first introduced. Primarily, the focus of telemedicine during the early days was on ensuring accessibility in remote and underserved regions, including rural areas, isolated communities, and environments where traditional medical facilities were not available. The

S. Siddiqui et al., *Connected Health Insights for Sustainable Development*,
https://doi.org/10.1007/978-3-031-81433-4_4

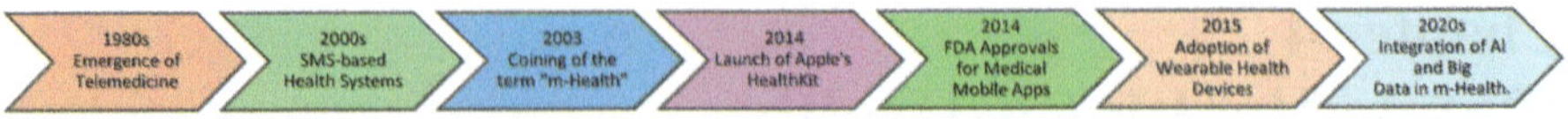

Fig. 4.1 Timeline for evolution of m-Health

major communication methods used for telemedicine were telephone, radio and fax machines; telephones were used for physician consultations, fax machines were used for transmitting medical records, and radio and television was used for awareness programs broadcast.

During 2000s, SMS-based health messaging services were introduced: health tips and preventive health advisory were sent to the patients' mobile phones; emergency alerts were sent during health crisis or disasters for ensuring the users' safety; appointment reminders were sent by clinics to reduce the no-show rates; similarly, medication reminders were sent to improve adherence, as well as health campaigns were also run via SMS for promoting the vaccination drives.

In 2003, Professor Robert Istepanian first coined the term "m-health" and defined it as "emerging mobile communications and network technologies for healthcare". Although transmission of preventive information and medication/appointment alerts had already begun with SMS based systems, the m-health opened up the new era of mobile applications and continuous health monitoring. The patients could now also consult their doctors using videoconferencing, which not only improved the quality of healthcare services but also significantly influenced the patients' behavior by supporting behavior change interventions through multimedia content, gamification, and personalized feedback.

In 2014, new opportunities in terms of health history management and trend monitoring developed with the launch of Apple HealthKit, which was a robust framework introduced to serve iOS ecosystem. The objective of this launch was to offer a centralized repository for health and fitness data; with this, users become able to maintain all their health records at one place. One of the key features of Healthkit was its possibility to share data with other applications: it offers a very high level of flexibility and abstraction to the developers as Healthkit offers a powerful API [2]. It also ensures the user privacy as any application connecting to it asks for the user's permission for reading or writing their data.

U.S. Food and Drug Administration (FDA) began to regularize the health-related mobile apps in 2014. FDA is responsible for protecting public health by ensuring the safety, efficacy, and security of drugs, biological products, and medical devices. With the advent of mobile health technology, the FDA extended its oversight to include mobile medical applications that could impact patient health. FDA recognized the importance of mobile apps, as it states "Mobile apps can help people manage their own health and wellness, promote healthy living, and gain access to useful information when and where they need it." [3]. The purpose of issuing approvals for mobile apps was not only to ensure patients' safety and confidence, but also to provide a guideline for the future developers about the components required in such apps. An example app that got approval during the early period is Mobile MIM app [4], which allowed doctors to view medical images like X-rays and MRIs on their

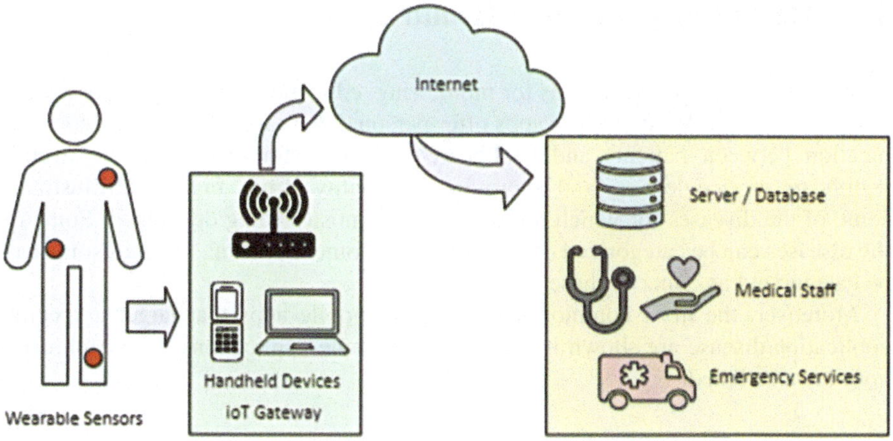

Fig. 4.2 Basic architecture of m-Health system

mobile devices. Similarly, another example is AliveCor Heart Monitor [5], which allowed users to record and monitor their heart rhythms using a mobile device. FDA approvals also increased the innovation rate for healthcare mobile apps as the developers had a clear pathway.

By 2015, the scope of m-health enhanced beyond mobile apps as the use of wearable devices gained popularity. The wearable devices connect with smart phones via communication standards such as Bluetooth and offered accessibility, independence and activity tracking via using smart sensors [6]. The patients, as a result, may get detailed health insights, customized treatments and long-term management at a reduced cost. Due to the regular monitoring, the wearables devices can inform the patients and physicians about the efficacy of ongoing treatment as well. The wearables are not only used for self-management by patients, but healthcare facilities also adopt these at a large-scale for better patient management and resource optimization. A typical m-Health architecture has been illustrated in Fig. 4.2, where the data goes from patient to the internet, and subsequently stored at the servers, and shared with the medical experts and emergency services.

2020s is the era where Artificial Intelligence and big data have been integrated with m-health to further enhance the health services. First, these technologies provide an opportunity to analyze vast amounts of data from various sources (like electronic health records, wearable devices, and genetic information) to provide personalized treatment plans, leading to better outcomes and more effective treatments. Second, AI models significantly help in preventive care as they predict disease outbreaks, patient deterioration, and potential health risks based on historical data and real-time monitoring. Early diagnosis and intervention also become possible due to the AI's capability of analyzing medical images such as MRIs, Xrays with high accuracy.

4.3 Major Categories of m-Health Apps

Mobile apps today, provide tools for monitoring, education, and support for a wide range of diseases. Most of these apps offer personalized care and facilitate communication between patients and healthcare providers, for enhancing the overall healthcare service delivery and improving the quality of life. Figure 4.3 illustrates some of the diseases for which mobile apps are mostly being developed. Some of the diseases can be categorized as physiological, some as mental, whereas some can be categorized as either of these.

Moreover, the most common categories of mobile apps that target a specific application/disease are shown in Table 4.1. Example applications from each category are also listed.

4.4 Achieving SDG 3 Through m-Health

As the focus of SDG 3 is on providing accessible healthcare for all at every age, m-health can certainly help to achieve it. For each of the targets and means of implementation detailed in Sects. 1.6 and 1.7, m-Health offers the relevant solution. Some of the ways in which m-Health contributes to achieving SDG3 are listed in Fig. 4.4, and discussed next.

4.4.1 Ensuring Healthcare Accessibility and Quality

First and foremost, m-Health solutions focus on making the healthcare accessible to everyone. Majority of the platforms not only allow remote monitoring, but also offer remote consultations, mostly valuable for the people from rural communities,

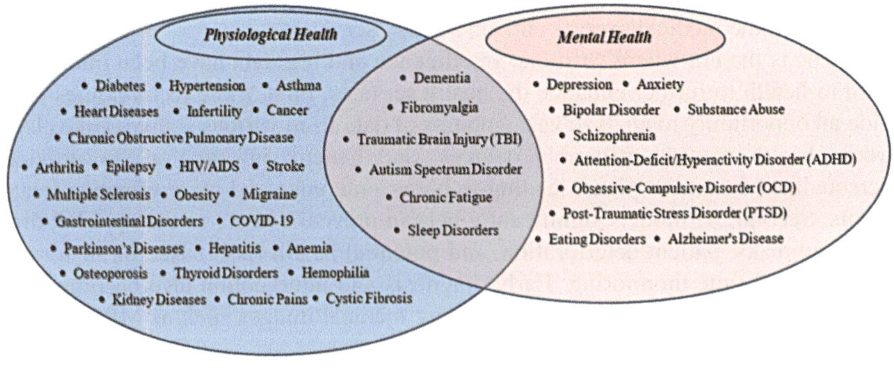

Fig. 4.3 Diseases treated by mobile apps

Table 4.1 Categories, purpose and examples of apps used for m-health

S. no	Category	Purpose	Example apps
1	Fitness and wellness tracking	Exercise tracking and diet monitoring.	MyFitnessPal, Fitbit
		Weight loss tracking and dietary guidance.	Lose It!, Noom
		Step counting and fitness tracking.	Pacer, Withings Health Mate
		Quick and effective workout routines.	7 Minute Workout
		Personalized coaching on lifestyle choices.	Fabulous, Lifesum
2	Remote monitoring	Continuous monitoring of patients' vital signs and chronic conditions.	Glucose Buddy, Cardiogram
		Symptom assessment and healthcare guidance.	Ada, iTriage
3	Telemedicine	Virtual consultations with doctors.	Doctor on Demand, Amwell
		Finding doctors and booking appointments.	Zocdoc, Heal
		Managing medications and reminders.	Medisafe, Mango Health
4	Medical reference and information	Medical reference and drug information.	Epocrates, WebMD
5	Mental health	Mental health support and mindfulness exercises.	Calm, Headspace, BetterHelp, Shine, Moodpath
		Supporting cognitive function and mental agility.	Lumosity, CogniFit
		Supporting behavioral change for better health outcomes.	Lark Health, Omada Health
		Online therapy and counseling.	Talkspace, BetterHelp
		Managing self-harm urges and providing mental health support.	Calm Harm
		12-week psychotherapy intervention for suicide prevention	WellPATH
		Manages employees' mental health	Whatsup?
		Self-assessment opportunity for health state	Interaktor
6	Chronic disease management	Blood pressure tracking and management.	SmartBP, Simple
		Diabetes logbook and blood sugar tracking.	MySugr, Glucose Buddy
		Heart rate monitoring and health tracking.	Cardiogram, AliveCor
		Mobile ECG and heart health tracking.	Kardia, AliveCor

(continued)

Table 4.1 (continued)

S. no	Category	Purpose	Example apps
7	Women's health	Tracking menstrual cycles, ovulation and reproductive health.	Clue, Ovia, Flo, Period Tracker by GP Apps
		Pregnancy tracking and infant care information.	Pregnancy+, BabyCenter
8	Substance abuse	Managing and overcoming addiction.	Leafly
		Support for quitting smoking.	Quit Genius
9	Allergy management	Tracking and managing allergies.	Allergy Alert
10	Sleep health	Monitoring sleep patterns and improving sleep quality.	Sleep Cycle, Aura
11	Hearing	Hearing tests.	hearScreen USA
12	Vision	Vision exercises.	EyeQue
		Tracking and improving vision health.	GlassesOff, VisioCare
13	Health information management	Managing health information and medications.	CareZone, Withings Health Mate
14	Child and infant care	Health tracking and information for children.	BlueLoop
15	Dental health	Dental care tracking and reminders.	iDental
16	Relaxation and meditation	Sleep and relaxation support.	Aura, Calm
17	Emergency services	First aid information and emergency response.	First Aid by American Red Cross
		Quick access to emergency medical services and instructions.	First Aid by American Red Cross
		On-demand house calls from doctors.	Heal
18	Environmental health	Monitoring environmental factors like air quality.	AirVisual, Plume Labs
19	Genetic information	Genetic testing information and personalized health advice.	23andMe, MyHeritage
20	Infectious disease tracking	Tracking outbreaks and providing information on infectious diseases.	HealthMap, Outbreaks Near Me
21	Occupational health	Improving health and safety in the workplace.	Ergonomics, Workplace Stress Tracker
22	Travel health	Health information and vaccination requirements for travelers.	CDC TravWell, TravelSmart
23	Pharmacy and medication delivery	Ordering medications and managing prescription deliveries.	PillPack, Capsule
		Comparing prescription drug prices and finding discounts.	GoodRx
24	Health communities	Connecting patients for support and information sharing.	PatientsLikeMe, Inspire, TalkLife
25	Clinical decision support	Assisting clinicians in making informed decisions.	VisualDx, Isabel Healthcare
26	Rehabilitation	Supporting physical rehabilitation and recovery.	PT Pal Pro, PhysioTech

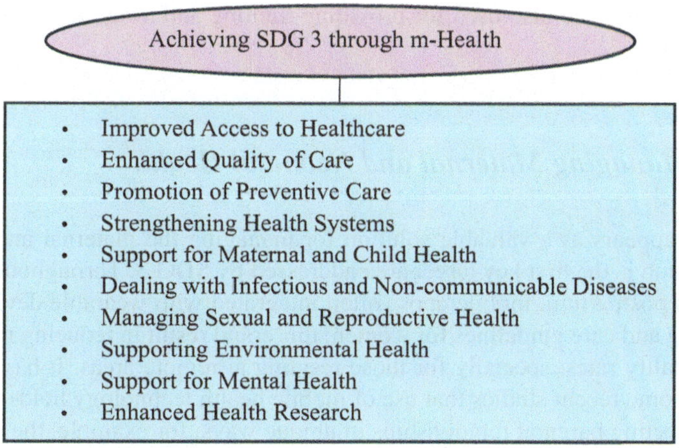

Fig. 4.4 Support of m-Health for SDG 3

who do not have such facilities otherwise. Similarly, m-Health platforms are widely used for raising health awareness. Secondly, the use of wearable devices in conjunction with mobile apps provide the advantages of continuous monitoring and medical recordkeeping; this leads to efficient management of chronic diseases. The quality of care delivered via m-Health has also been subsequently enhanced due to the use of AI and big data; now the professionals are able to drive detailed insights about patients' health and make informed decisions accordingly. In addition to collecting data from various sources, m-Health platforms also improve adherence to medicine and other medical advice. As indicated previously in Table 4.1, various mobile apps offer reminders for medications, exercise schedules, doctor appointments etc. Furthermore, preventive care has become possible as AI driven tools create personalized health and fitness plans based on individual data.

4.4.2 Strengthening Health Systems

Health resource management is another key area targeted by m-Health. Use of m-Health technologies reduce the cost, improves the resource utilization and reduces inefficiencies. Due to the continuous use of m-Health platforms, the need for physical clinic visits reduces, which in turn reduces the healthcare burden on clinical facilities and state budget; hence, the available physicians can manage more patients while maintaining the quality of care. Similarly, hospitalizations and emergency interventions also reduce as patients are continuously monitored and preventive strategies are in place. The administrative tasks are streamlined as patients are increasingly relying on m-Health platforms for scheduling appointments; the automated scheduling reduces the hassles of queuing as well as the need of extensive administrative staff. Moreover, m-Health platforms are not only beneficial for the patients, but they are also used for providing training and awareness to the healthcare workers.

4.4.3 Managing Maternal and Neonatal Health

m-Health appears as a valuable solution for managing the maternal and neonatal health, which is the first key target area addressed by SDG 3. Throughout the pregnancy and postpartum, mobile apps (often integrated with wearable devices) offer monitoring and care guidelines for women; this could result in reducing mother and child mortality rates, specially for those residing at remote areas. It has also been found by some recent studies that use of mobile health technology holds the potential for affecting parental relationships in unique ways; for example, the pregnancy apps mediate the mother's relationship with her unborn child, the parents' awareness about the pregnant body and sharing of experience between the partners [7]. Similarly, for new born and older children, mobile apps help parents to track the

Table 4.2 AI for fetal health monitoring

S. no.	AI algorithm	Fetal abnormality monitored
1	Convolutional Neural Networks (CNN)	Congenital heart defects
2	Support Vector Machines (SVM)	Neural tube defects
3	Random Forests	Chromosomal abnormalities (e.g., Down syndrome)
4	U-Net	Fetal growth restriction
5	ResNet	Fetal echocardiography analysis
6	Recurrent Neural Networks (RNN)	Abnormal fetal heart rate patterns
7	Logistic Regression	Preterm birth prediction
8	Decision Trees	Placental abnormalities
9	k-Nearest Neighbors (k-NN)	Fetal distress detection
10	Gradient Boosting Machines (GBM)	Intrauterine growth restriction (IUGR)
11	Bayesian Networks	Risk assessment for fetal abnormalities
12	Genetic Algorithms	Prediction of genetic disorders
13	Artificial Neural Networks (ANN)	Detection of fetal alcohol syndrome
14	Ensemble Methods (e.g., XGBoost)	Comprehensive fetal health monitoring
15	Principal Component Analysis (PCA)	Dimensionality reduction in fetal anomaly detection
16	Reinforcement Learning	Optimization of monitoring protocols
17	Autoencoders	Anomaly detection in fetal ultrasound images
18	Clustering Algorithms (e.g., K-Means)	Grouping of fetal abnormalities for analysis

vaccination schedules, be aware about the disease outbreaks and monitor their children' growth milestones.

Moreover, there have been AI-powered m-Health solutions developed to inform the parents and caregivers about any diseases or abnormality in the fetus [8]. Table 4.2 lists some of the common AI algorithms that can be used to detect specific fetal abnormality.

4.4.4 Dealing with Infectious and Noncommunicable Diseases

m-Health tools have been used for various use cases related to infectious diseases. During the recent surge of COVID-19, hundreds of mobile apps were used and developed for real-time disease surveillance and outbreak tracking, enabling quick responses to infectious disease threats. Some of the most common uses of mobile apps during COVID-19 are listed in Fig. 4.5. Starting from collecting symptoms and reminding to wash hands, there were apps that offered mental support using community building and alternative medicine techniques such as music therapy [9]. The mobile apps are also used for conducting awareness campaigns during infectious disease outbreaks; hence, m-health could reduce the rate of disease spread as well as anxiety and depression caused by it.

m-health platforms have also been offering great assistance to patients with chronic (non-communicable) diseases. Wearable technology has been used at homes and hospitals to ensure that patients vitals are maintained within healthy limits. The chronic conditions such as hypertension, asthma, diabetes, heart diseases and can easily be managed via m-health platforms, reducing the healthcare costs and improving the quality of life. As discussed above, mobile health apps provide tools for tracking vital signs, medication reminders, and lifestyle management, empowering patients to take an active role in their own care. Moreover, through the

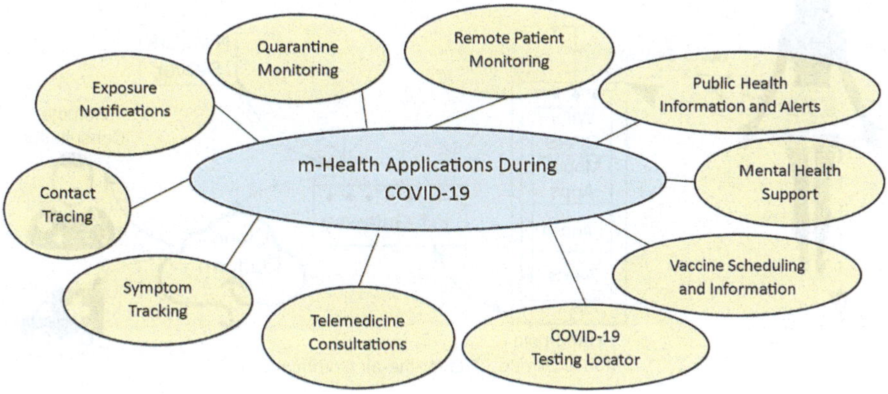

Fig. 4.5 Applications of m-Health during COVID-19 epidemic

integration of AI and big data, patients as well as their physicians are informed about the health risks; in this regard, various health monitoring dashboards have been developed in order to providing customized risk tracking for patients [10]. With the help of AI-powered dashboards, personalized treatment strategies and timely interventions are become possible.

4.4.5 Managing Sexual and Reproductive Health

As indicated in Table 4.2, there are various mobile applications specifically developed for menstrual period or fertility monitoring. These apps offer women a convenient way to track their menstrual cycles, ovulation, and fertility windows. Most of these apps use data input by users, such as period start and end dates, symptoms, and basal body temperature, to predict future cycles and fertile days. Some apps are also being proposed to be connected to implanted sensors, for a better monitoring of ovulation. An example architecture of m-health platform integrating implanted sensors for fertility monitoring, is shown in Fig. 4.6. Here, the nano-sensors will collect data from the Fallopian tubes, and would communicate by using THz and molecular communication links within the human body to transmit the information to the on-body device; subsequently, the information about presence of eggs/any disease etc. shall be transmitted to hand-held device using conventional means of Bluetooth/ WiFi/5G. this way, information about the fertility window or any disease could be timely communicated, ensuring the health of women and their future children.

Many of the fertility monitoring apps also provide educational content on reproductive health, reminders for taking medications or supplements, and personalized health insights. By leveraging these tools, women can better understand their bodies, plan for pregnancy, and manage conditions like polycystic ovary syndrome

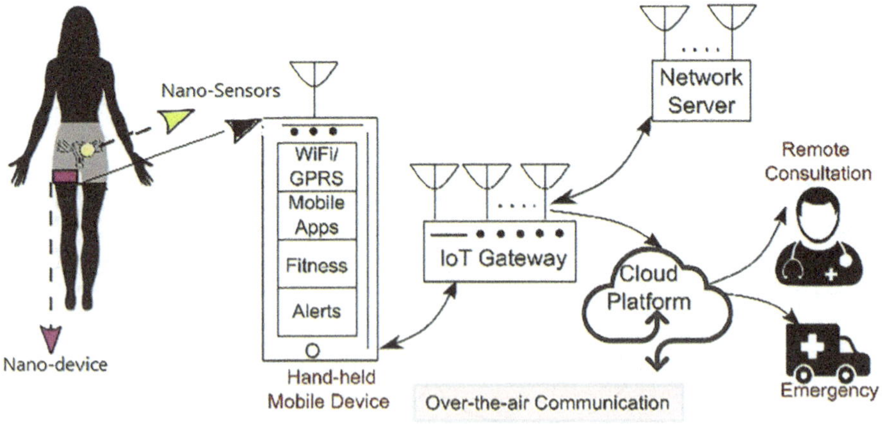

Fig. 4.6 A hybrid m-Health architecture for fertility monitoring using implanted sensor nodes

(PCOS) or irregular periods. The community support is also available on most of the fertility apps so the women may learn from each others' experiences, share their emotions and have a sense of relatability and support. These platforms provide forums and chat groups where users can share their personal stories, seek advice, and offer encouragement leading to a better experience, whether a woman is going through challenging phase of conceiving a child, menopause or even fighting with various types of cancers.

4.4.6 Monitoring Environmental Health

m-Health solutions also assist the user in managing their health based on the environmental data. Most health apps, in addition to collecting vital data, also collect information about environment such as air quality, temperature, humidity, and other environmental parameters in real-time. Based on this information, the users are kept informed about any environmental hazards, pollution levels, unsafe water conditions, or chemical spills. To facilitate the movement and activities of users, m-Health apps also integrate GPS for identifying the hazardous locations. For example, the users while planning their day-out or exercise may consult their app to check the pollution level and choose the locations accordingly. In addition to the routine environmental monitoring for aiding individual users, m-Health apps also have a potential to collect information from satellite for having an insight into large-scale environmental state. Deforestation, urban sprawl, and changes in water bodies for various locations can be identified; such information is intended to help the users to plan their movement/activities, and also to the state for managing their environmental conservation efforts and urban development strategies effectively.

The deployment of environmental data by the m-Health apps also opens new dimensions of health research. The environmental data, in its association of impact on public health can be assessed, leading to identification of correlation between these. For example, it is well-known that there is a correlation between environmental pollution and respiratory diseases; however, using mobile sensing technologies and apps, it becomes possible to quantify the impact of pollution on patients belonging from various age groups, disease history etc. Similarly, health risks, and outbreaks can also be predicted. Hence, the prevention strategies can be planned much more effectively.

4.4.7 Support for Mental Health

m-Health has significantly broadened the scope of mental healthcare. Despite having serious affects, mental health is not often prioritized. There are various factors responsible for their ignorance including lack of awareness, accessibility and resources. Moreover, in many cultures, seeking mental health assistance is a taboo

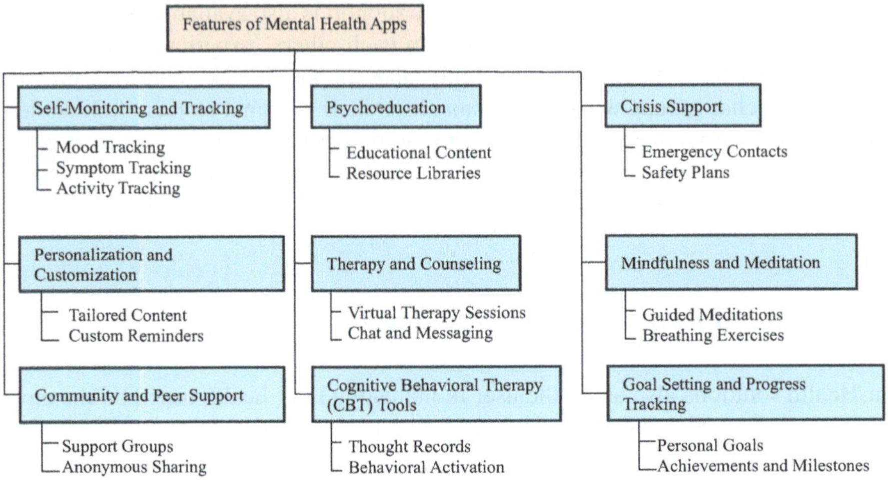

Fig. 4.7 Managing mental health via m-Health apps

as yet, which also causes hinderances in accessing assessment and therapy services. Through the use of m-Health platforms, users get an opportunity of getting their mental health assessed, and monitored on a continuous basis, while eliminating the associated stigma. Various apps offer remote video consultations which reduces the need for physical clinical visits, making the process cost effective and accessible. Hence, the use of m-Health solutions bridges gaps in traditional mental health services, ensuring more people receive the care they need, which is a direct contribution to SDG 3.

There are also a large number of services that are offered by mental health apps, and platforms that integrate wearable devices for continuous assessment of issues such as anxiety and depression. A basic taxonomy indicating the features offered by common mental health apps/platforms is illustrated in Fig. 4.7:

4.5 Enhancing Health Research

Due to the enormous data generated by m-Health apps and platforms, novel opportunities for improving health outcomes through research have been developed. m-health has enabled continuous data collection. For example, earlier the data about blood pressure, blood sugar, heart rate, sleep patterns etc. was only recorded when the patients used to visit the clinical facilities; also, the scope of this data was limited to only the patients who could visit. Now with the advent of m-health, the data may be collected several times a day not only from the regular patients who have physical access to the clinics, but also from those who reside at far-off locations and could not get their data recorded. There are multiple sources of data entry, wearable devices using communication standards such as Bluetooth, clinical information systems, patient surveys, pharmacy information systems, ambient home sensors, etc. Moreover, data from users' social media accounts is also often integrated with the m-health apps. Hence, the volume of data has increased exponentially which facilitates health research in the areas of enhanced predictive modeling, personalized medicine, population health management, resource management, drug discovery and development and real-time response strategies.

4.6 Challenges and Opportunities

Figure 4.8 presents a framework indicating the major challenges and future opportunities associated with m-Health, highlighting key factors that influence the implementation and impact of mobile health technologies. Let's briefly discuss each of these.

4.7 Key Challenges

4.7.1 Technology Integration

This appears as one of the most critical and immediate challenge for wide-scale global adoption of m-Health. For decades, there have been manual systems used for health data management; now, mobile technology requires the stakeholders to integrate novel solutions with the existing conventional healthcare systems. Many healthcare providers use diverse and even outdated electronic health record (EHR) systems, making interoperability a complex issue. Ensuring that mobile health applications and devices can seamlessly exchange data with these systems requires robust standardization and cooperation among technology providers. Without effective integration, the potential benefits of m-Health, such as real-time data sharing

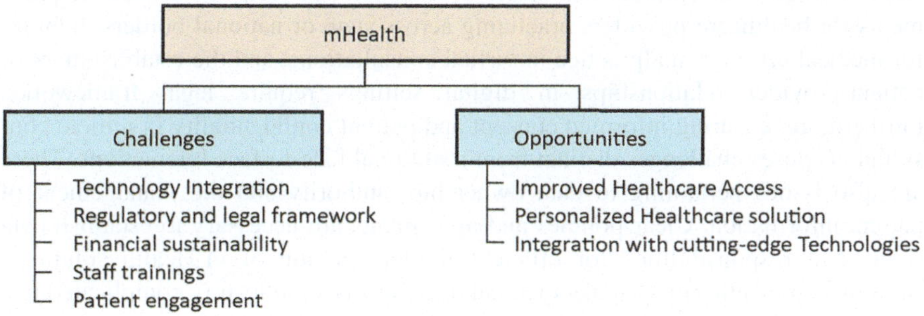

Fig. 4.8 Framework presenting challenges and opportunities of m-Health

and comprehensive patient records, cannot be fully realized, leading to inefficiencies.

Another major concern is to ensure privacy and security while using m-health platforms. These solutions deal with highly personal and sensitive information, which is stored and transmitted over mobile devices, cloud or both. The extensive usage of patient information does not only create security threats for individuals but also for hospitals. For example, a patient expects the clinical information system to provide access so they may schedule appointments, access their health trends, download their reports etc. which clearly increases security threats, by creating more possibilities of intrusion. Ensuring the Confidentiality, Integrity, and Availability (CIA) of this data requires robust encryption methods, secure communication protocols, and stringent access controls. Despite these measures, mobile health applications remain vulnerable to cyberattacks, data breaches, and unauthorized access, which can erode trust among users and healthcare providers. Therefore, ongoing efforts to enhance cybersecurity measures and comply with regulatory standards, such as HIPAA in the United States, are essential to safeguard patient information.

Finally, regardless of how advanced or useful a m-Health app may be, it always needs a reliable and secure internet connection to be fully functional. Most of these applications either focus on storing patient's data on cloud, or telemedicine facilities. As of present, many rural and far-off areas lack even the basic internet infrastructure which could hinder the use of these apps. If the use of m-Health apps become more prevalent, the presence of digital divide would affect the accessibility to healthcare facilities even more. Addressing this challenge involves investing in telecommunications infrastructure, exploring alternative connectivity solutions such as satellite internet, and developing offline functionalities for mobile health applications to ensure continuous care in the remote areas.

4.7.2 Regulatory and Legal Framework

Due to the unique nature of m-Health, novel legal requirements have surfaced, in contrast to the conventional healthcare settings. Issues such as licensure requirements for healthcare providers practicing across state or national borders, liability for medical errors or malpractice in virtual consultations, and the establishment of patient-provider relationships in digital settings require legal frameworks. Furthermore, ensuring informed consent and patient confidentiality in remote consultations poses challenges distinct from traditional face-to-face interactions. There are also issues pertaining to data ownership, authority and the management of patient information. Clear policies and agreements are necessary to establish data rights and responsibilities for efficient implementation of m-Health solutions. Moreover, the authority to make medical decisions is significantly complicated in a remote context, especially for the cases where multiple healthcare providers are involved.

For ensuring efficient and ethical clinical practices while using mobile technologies, it is crucial to comply with the regulatory frameworks discussed above. Since the technology of m-Health is still in infancy, it is a major challenge to integrate the regulatory guidelines of different countries/regions and different healthcare sectors. For example, each country and healthcare organization may have distinct laws and standards concerning aspects of patient privacy, data protection, medical device certification, and telemedicine practices. Also, lack of awareness and expertise of medical professionals with the legal requirements may cause hinderance in ethical and legal implementation of m-Health solutions. Failure to adhere to these regulations can result in fines, or even the suspension of m-Health services. Therefore, a collaboration of legal and medical experts is often required to ensure smooth and efficient implementation of m-Health.

4.7.3 Financial Sustainability

Since the technology of m-Health is in infancy at most places globally, it is not intuitive to prove the financial sustainability. Evaluation of financial sustainability of m-Health systems actually needs comparison with the conventional healthcare systems. Although, theoretically m-Health promises to lower the healthcare costs by reducing the needs of physical clinical visits, improving the preventive care etc., it does require initial investments to build m-Health infrastructure, train the staff, developing legal frameworks and raising patient awareness. Moreover, the cost-savings can be demonstrated by conducting longitudinal studies and public health surveys, which have not yet been realized.

There are also issues related to compensation of medical staff providing m-Health services. Since there are no relevant regulations developed so far, there is significant variability among mobile apps in terms of compensation for services such as tele-consultations, remote monitoring, and digital therapeutics. Also, there is yet a lack of clarity regarding reimbursement of insurance claims made for services availed via m-Health platforms; this lack of standardized reimbursement policies can discourage healthcare providers from adopting m-Health solutions [11]. Thus, there is a need for relevant stakeholders to devise efficient compensation and reimbursement policies governing the m-Health transactions.

4.7.4 Staff Trainings

The maximum potential of m-Health technologies can only be achieved by providing trainings to the healthcare staff. In the m-Health architecture shown in Fig. 4.2, medical experts are the key stakeholders responsible for integrating the m-Health technologies with healthcare systems. They monitor the patient conditions, manage the health trends and make key decisions regarding diagnostics, treatments or procedures. To ensure smooth operation of m-Health solutions, it is required that medical staff is comfortable with the use of common tools such ash smart phone applications, wearable devices, centralized dashboards and clinical information systems. Due to the diversity of the m-Health devices and systems, continuous training and education is required for keeping them updated with the latest technology trends.

In addition to offering the technical guidance, the medical staff also need to be trained for the revised information flows and patient management. With the integration of m-Health solutions, the key processes and ways using which the staff interacted with patients has changed. Now, the patients are empowered and clinical workflows are mostly aligned with the patients' preferences offering the utmost flexibility which is the unique feature of m-Health. Hence, Empowering healthcare professionals with the knowledge and skills to motivate and support patients in using m-Health tools can significantly improve patient outcomes and satisfaction.

4.7.5 Patient Engagement

As the primary goal of m-Health is to provide accessibility to a broad range of users, one of the main challenges is developing user-friendly interfaces that cater to diverse populations. Personalized and user-friendly interfaces can significantly enhance the patients' experience, making it easier for them to integrate m-Health tools into their daily routines. Just like the staff trainings, there is also a need to conduct awareness and education programs for patients, which should provide enough confidence to the patients for taking charge of their own health. Also, offering a chance of sharing concerns regarding m-Health experience with the medical experts improves patients' engagement. Moreover, regular feedback and support, such as through reminders, progress tracking, and virtual check-ins, help maintain patient motivation and adherence.

4.8 Key Opportunities

m-Health presents numerous opportunities to revolutionize healthcare delivery by enhancing accessibility, personalizing care, and improving health outcomes. Let's discuss some of these briefly.

4.8.1 Improved Healthcare Access

First, m-Health offers opportunity for improved healthcare access for patients belonging from far-off locations as it attempts at eliminating the needs for physical visits. The patients can benefit from remote monitoring and consultations, particularly for chronic health conditions where data can be entered via numerous sources including patient reported questionnaires as well as wearable devices. The emergence of new sensing technologies also provides an opportunity of timely prediction of the diseases, which could have gone unnoticed otherwise; for example, a range of optical sensors has been developed for identifying Diabetes and cardiovascular conditions [12].

The use of m-Health platforms also reduces costs through enabling timely medical interventions, which lowers the burden on healthcare facilities and state. Furthermore, due to the continuous monitoring, the need of readmissions also reduces which helps the medical facilities to deal with more patients. The chances of effective coordination and collaboration between physicians belonging from various locations also improve due to m-Health: the real-time data streams as well as all the previous history of patient can be shared quickly through m-Health apps.

4.8.2 Personalized Health Solutions

m-Health offers an opportunity to develop highly personalized treatment plans based on the real-time data. Unlike the conventional healthcare systems, where the treatment could only be modified once the patient visited the clinic and either reported their symptoms or their vitals were measured using ordinary devices. Now, the vital parameters data is continuously transmitted to the medical experts in the real-time; this data transmission helps the doctors to make any change in the treatment/medication plan without even the need of patient to visit the clinic. Similarly, there are apps which monitor the impact of medication on the patient's vitals; this information is continuously shared with the doctors, who could devise a personalized treatment plan to foster a more proactive approach to healthcare.

Predictive analytics is another technique offered by m-Health where large datasets generated from real-time health monitoring activities are analyzed. Based on these analytics, correlations, patterns, and potential health risks can be identified in the patients even before they show symptoms. This proactive approach allows for early intervention and preventive measures, improving outcomes and potentially saving lives.

4.8.3 Integration with Cutting-Edge Technologies

Integration of m-Health with advanced computing techniques of Artificial intelligence and Big Data Analytics has exponentially enhanced the scope of remote health management. AI algorithms can process vast amounts of health data collected through m-Health devices, identifying patterns and generating insights that would be impossible for humans to detect manually. For example, machine learning models can predict patient outcomes and suggest personalized treatment plans based on individual health data, continuously learning and improving as more data is collected. Big Data Analytics further enables the aggregation and analysis of massive datasets from diverse sources, including electronic health records, wearable devices, and patient-reported outcomes. For example, big data techniques can reveal population health trends, track the spread of infectious diseases, and identify risk factors for chronic conditions. The integration of these advanced computing techniques with m-Health facilitates real-time decision-making, predictive analytics and personalized medicine, empowering healthcare providers to deliver timely and effective interventions.

References

1. Word Health Organization (WHO), Document A71: mHealth—Use of appropriate digital technologies for public health. PLoS Med. **10**(1) (2018)
2. What is Healthkit. Accessed 02 July 2024. [Online]. Available: https://cocoacasts.com/what-is-healthkit
3. Device Software Functions Including Mobile Medical Applications I FDA. Accessed 02 July 2024. [Online]. Available: https://www.fda.gov/medical-devices/digital-health-center-excellence/device-software-functions-including-mobile-medical-applications
4. Mobile MIM™ I Portable Diagnostic Imaging for iOS and MacOS. Accessed 02 July 2024. [Online]. Available: https://www.mimsoftware.com/remote-access/mobile-mim
5. ECG Monitor I Viatom Technology Co. Accessed 02 July 2024. [Online]. Available: https://www.viatomtech.com/ecgmonitor
6. R. LeMoyne, T. Mastroianni, Evolutions for wearable and wireless systems, in *Smart Sensors, Measurement and Instrumentation*, (Springer, Singapore, 2024), pp. 135–147. https://doi.org/10.1007/978-981-97-2439-0_12
7. C. Eliasson, Pregnancy apps: The birth of a new experience: Exploring the entangled relationship between pregnant people and pregnancy apps (2024). Accessed 03 July 2024. [Online]. Available: https://urn.kb.se/resolve?urn=urn:nbn:se:uu:diva-533133
8. A. Shiwlani et al., Prediction of fetal brain and heart abnormalties using artificial intelligence algorithms: A review. Am. J. Biomed. Sci. Res. **22**(3) (2024). https://doi.org/10.34297/AJBSR.2024.22.002970
9. S. Siddiqui, A.A. Khan, F. Nait-Abdesselam, I. Dey, Anxiety and depression management for elderly using Internet of Things and symphonic melodies. IEEE Int. Conf. Commun. (2021). https://doi.org/10.1109/ICC42927.2021.9500419
10. S. Siddiqui, F. Nait-Abdesselam, A.A. Khan, I. Dey, Enabling real-time dashboards for anxiety risk classification using the internet of things, in *Proceedings—IEEE Global Communications Conference, GLOBECOM*, (2021). https://doi.org/10.1109/GLOBECOM46510.2021.9685683
11. M. Addotey-Delove, R.E. Scott, M. Mars, Healthcare workers' perspectives of mHealth adoption factors in the developing world: Scoping review. Int. J. Environ. Res. Public Health **20**(2) (2023). https://doi.org/10.3390/ijerph20021244
12. E.A. Zherebtsov et al., Wireless dynamic light scattering sensors detect microvascular changes associated with ageing and diabetes. IEEE Trans. Biomed. Eng. **70**(11) (2023). https://doi.org/10.1109/TBME.2023.3275654

Chapter 5
Personalized Medicine

5.1 Limitations of Traditional Medicine

By design, the traditional medicine is focused on treating symptoms and disease rather than prevention. There are various limitations of the traditional medicine, due to which their effectiveness may be compromised. First and foremost, the traditional medicine takes one-size fits all approach; often the standardized treatment protocols and medication dosages are set based on the results obtained from broad clinical trials. Although, the participants for such clinical trails are selected using specific sampling strategies, the resulting outcomes may not be relevant for every individual due to differences in lifestyle, genetics and environment. Secondly, the objective of the standardized treatments is to treat and average patient; as a result, the subtle differences among patient profiles may result in side effects.

Thirdly, there is no consideration of monitoring patient's response to the medicine in the traditional medicine; the physicians recommend a dosage based on the patient's condition, history and physician's own past practice and evidence-based research; however, the patient's response to the medicine is not monitored, which could be different for everyone due to their genetic, metabolic and other attributes. Now in case the patient develops some reaction or side effect after taking a dose or two, there is no monitoring and control to stop/alter the treatment right away. Hence, a delay is naturally involved in the processes of diagnostics and treatment, as the patients generally report after completing one failed cycle of medication. The situation might become critical if traditional medicine leads to adverse effects such as toxicity for some patients. Moreover, it is also challenging to manage the long-term chronic conditions by using traditional medicine.

S. Siddiqui et al., *Connected Health Insights for Sustainable Development*,
https://doi.org/10.1007/978-3-031-81433-4_5

5.2 How It Works?

The process of developing personalized medicine involves patients and their data is continuously collected for feedback and adjustment. A typical cycle of personalized medicine development and modification has been illustrated in Fig. 5.1. The first step in the process of personalized medicine development is data collection from the patient. The data about physiological parameters can be collected using wearable sensors; however, more invasive methods are used for collecting DNA samples and genetic information through blood, saliva and tissue samples. Moreover, genetic testing is also done for identifying unique genetic variations and mutations that may influence disease risk and drug response. Next, the obtained information is integrated together; for example, the genetic information is integrated with the data about previous diseases history, lifestyle and environmental factors. All of the available data is then assessed to develop a unique patient profile; this helps to identify the prevailing risks for each patient based on their genetic makeup and other factors. These predictions can be used for managing early interventions, such as suggesting lifestyle changes or taking a certain vitamin. Since the treatment plans are made highly tailored to an individual, the chances of side effects and treatment failure are reduced significantly as compared to traditional medicine.

The next step is to continuously monitor the patient's response to treatment through regular follow-ups and biomarker analysis. As shown in Fig. 5.1, this monitoring helps to identify the impact of treatment plan on the patient. Finally, feedback is generated and required improvement/modification is made in the treatment plan/ medicine development.

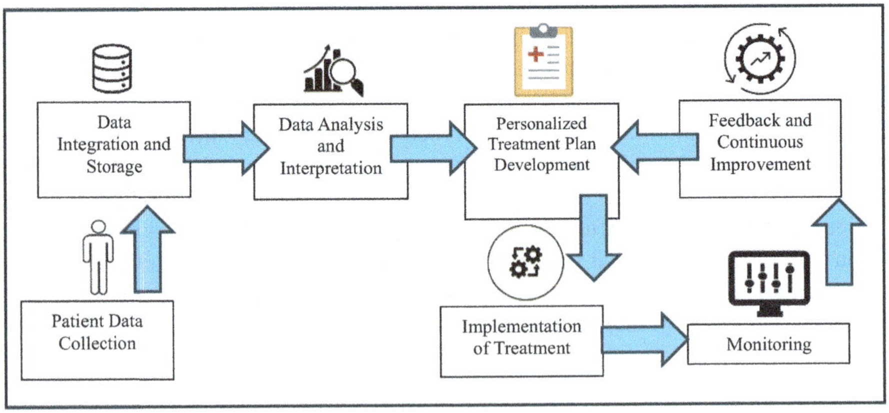

Fig. 5.1 Process of personalized medicine development and implementation

5.3 Factors Governing Personalized Medicine

There are several key factors that govern the successful development and implementation of personalized medicine. Some of these are personal, whereas others are external such as cultural and environmental. Let's briefly look at some of the most crucial factors:

5.3.1 Genetic Makeup

Unique genetic code of every patient can significantly impact their response to the medications. For example, Single nucleotide polymorphisms (SNPs) are common genetic variations that usually affects drug metabolism, efficacy, and the risk of side effects. Genetic variations can also affect the structure and function of drug targets (e.g., receptors, enzymes), altering the drug's effectiveness. Similarly, Copy Number Variations (CNVs) can also influence gene expression and can contribute to differences in disease susceptibility and drug response. The genetic makeup interacts with environmental factors which also influences the risk of diseases and outcomes of treatments. For example, individuals with certain genetic profiles might be more susceptible to environmental toxins, which can affect disease progression and response to therapies.

In addition, some genetic variations increase the risk of side effects and reactions. For example, variations in the HLA-B gene can predict severe hypersensitivity reactions to certain drugs, such as carbamazepine and abacavir. Testing for genetic makeup also helps to identify the mutations responsible for hereditary diseases such as those found in Huntington's disease (HTT gene) and cystic fibrosis (CFTR gene).

5.3.2 Medical History

Medical history plays a significant role to affect the process of medicine personalization. Since each patient has a unique medical history, it is used for developing customized treatment plans; for example, the medicines which have worked well in the past may be continued with the patients, while those which have caused allergic or other reactions could be avoided. The customized chronic disease management plans can also be developed based on the knowledge about previous history of diabetes, asthma or hypertension. Furthermore, having continuous monitoring and history management, it becomes possible to identify the trends of chronic disease prevention, which helps to modify the treatment plans in the correct direction. In addition to having the disease history, knowledge about lifestyle factors such as exercise routines, substance use and diet also helps to develop customized treatment and lifestyle recommendation plans.

Moreover, knowledge about patient's family history is also critical for personalized medicine. There are various diseases which are governed by the genetic predispositions including diabetes, heart diseases and cancer. If the automated system or physicians know about the family history, the patients can easily be advised for taking preventive measures, early interventions can also be planned. Similarly, relevant genetic testing may be conducted for patients with unique family histories; for example, individuals with a family history of breast or ovarian cancer might undergo BRCA1 and BRCA2 testing. Subsequently, the history also affects interpretation of genetic tests and distinguishing between pathogenic variants and benign ones.

5.3.3 *Lifestyle Factors*

Lifestyle factors highly motivate the need and development of personalized medicine, due to having a large influence of disease prevalence and medication efficiency. First and foremost, varying dietary habits significantly influence the disease risk, such as for diabetes and cardiovascular diseases. Similarly, fitness level and exercise routines affect the health outcomes. The substance use also affects the disease risks and treatment response; moreover, stress, sleep patterns also impact mental health. In addition to having an influence on the disease risk, activity level and diet also affect the treatment response and effectiveness. Based on the assessment of lifestyle factors, personalized medicine offers customized treatment strategies to mostly deal with the chronic conditions like hypertension, diabetes, and obesity.

Personalized medicine addresses the needs of individual by developing the intervention plans that align well with their lifestyle. For example, dietary recommendations and exercise plans are made based on an individual's genetic predispositions and lifestyle. Medicine dosages are adjusted to improve efficacy and reduce side effects for each patient based on their unique profile. Targeted screening programs are made using the risk profiles created after assessment of the patients' lifestyle data; this helps to achieve efficient risk assessment and ensure prevention and/or early intervention. Even efficient behavioral interventions can be designed using holistic data and medical history about each patient. Since the treatment plans are developed according to the lifestyle, the adherence is usually higher as compared to the conventional medication.

5.3.4 *Environmental Influences*

There are various environmental factors that encourage the development of personalized medicine as it could tailor the medication needs for individuals. The exposure to certain types of environments can lead people to various serious diseases;

therefore, knowing about the environmental risk factors for people can help to develop preventive strategies and customized medicine. For example, air and water pollution as well as soil contamination increase the risk of various diseases including certain types of cancers and, cardiovascular and respiratory diseases. Similarly, contaminants such as heavy metals and pesticides often present in water and soil can also affect health negatively.

The environmental factors related to climate and weather also pose significant risks for individuals, based on their unique vulnerabilities. Many of the environmental factors vary geographically and seasonally, encouraging the use of personalized medicine. Heat waves, extreme weather and exposure to allergens all can be dealt by developing personalized prevention and treatment strategies. Another prevailing issue of the present times is increased exposure of populations to natural, medical and occupational radiations. Exposure to natural radioactive gas radon increases the risk of lung cancer; similarly, people may be subject to high radiation exposure due to their occupations or medical treatment. For example, the workforce in certain factories/mines is exposed to numerous harmful chemicals and gases, often leading to serious health risks. As a matter of fact, routine exposure to household chemicals such as plastics, cleaning agents can also affect health. In all such cases, personalized monitoring is essential to ensure that the risks associated with radiation can be minimized for everyone.

In addition to pollutants and radiation exposure, the socio-economic and cultural factors also motivate the use of personalized medicine. Accessibility to healthcare and healthy lifestyle facilities is largely governed by the socio-economic status of people. Personalized medicine is based on the monitoring of these factors and offers customized healthcare solutions. Particularly, access to and awareness about mental health is very limited in the low-income groups and developing countries. The use of personalized medicine and associated technologies of IoT and AI help to improve the reach of mental healthcare. For example, online mental health assessment through survey questionnaires, and mobile apps has become common with various psychologists [1]. Affordable wearable devices are also playing a crucial role in remote monitoring and management of physical and mental health. Based on the data collected from patients and mobile apps, customized therapy sessions are conducted that fit to the needs of patients coming from diverse backgrounds.

5.4 Deploying IoT, AI and DS

Numerous techniques from the domains of IoT, AI and DS have been deployed for achieving the major goal of personalized medicine, i.e., to improve patient outcomes by improving the healthcare service delivery. This section sheds light on some of the emerging computing techniques, for their association with personalized medicine.

5.4.1 Wearable Devices

As previously discussed in Sect. 5.2, the first point of data collection for personalized medicine is the wearable devices. These devices collect data about various physiological parameters to facilitate continuous real-time tracking of patient's health state. Some of the major parameters that are being monitored using smart watches, fitness trackers and wi-fi/Bluetooth enabled devices include blood pressure, pulse rate, blood sugar, physical activity level, body temperature and others. Also, with the advancements in material sciences, the flexibility and stretchability of wearable devices/patches has increased. There are various categories of wearable sensors, as illustrated in Fig. 5.2.

The most common categories of wearable sensors include biometric, motion and activity, environmental, chemical/biochemical, respiratory, neurological, optical, pressure & force, temperature & humidity and multi-modal sensors. Let's briefly define each category below:

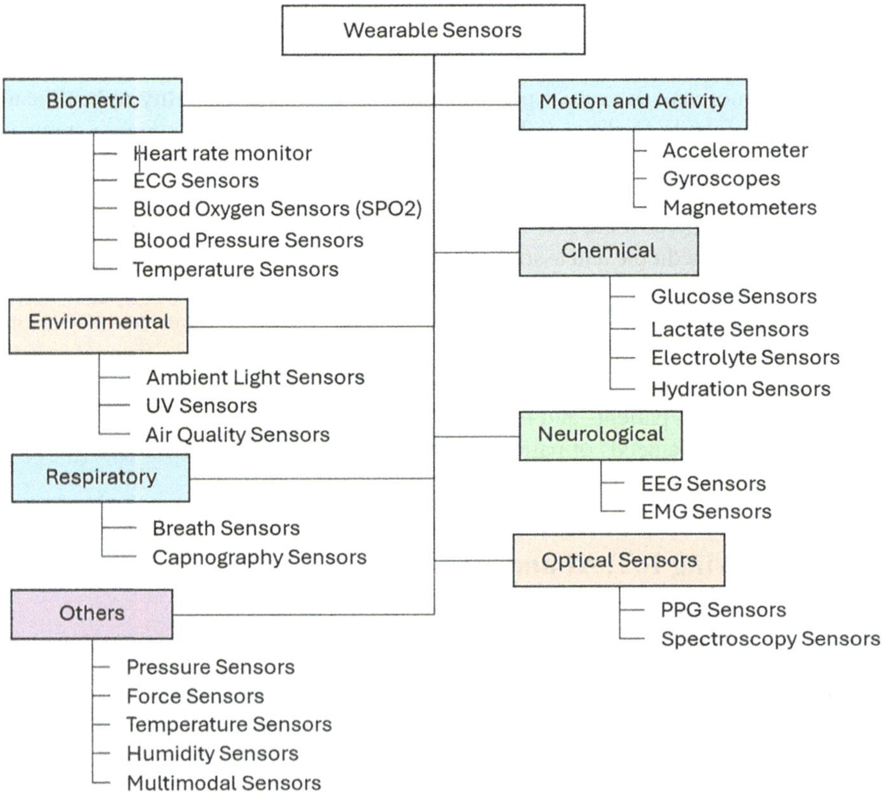

Fig. 5.2 Categories of wearable sensors

- From the biometric category, heart rate monitors, measure the heart rate using electrical or optical sensors. Electrocardiogram (ECG) sensors detect cardiac conditions such as arrhythmias by recording the electric activity. Blood Oxygen Sensors (SpO_2) sensors use pulse oximetry technique to measure blood oxygen levels. Blood Pressure Sensors use pressure-based or optical methods for tracking systolic and diastolic blood pressure. Temperature sensors monitor the body temperature either to detect fever or to detect fertility status by monitoring changes in the basal temperature.
- From the category of motion and activity sensors, accelerometers detect movement, activity levels and orientation by measuring acceleration. Gyroscopes provide data about orientation and balance by tracking rotational movements. Magnetometers are also used to detect orientation and direction; these are often used in combination with gyroscopes and accelerometers for having more precise and accurate information about motion.
- From environmental sensors category, ambient light sensors measure and help to regulate light intensity with a focus on regulating cardia rhythms and improving sleep quality. Ultraviolet (UV) sensors monitor exposure to UV light for prevention of skin damage. Similarly, air quality sensors detect allergens and pollutants present in the environment to guide the users about prevention strategies; these sensors often play a crucial role for managing diseases like asthma and developing customized treatment plans.
- From chemical and biochemical sensors category, Glucose sensors are often used for diabetic patients for continuous and/or remote monitoring of glucose levels. Lactate sensors are used to measure fatigue by detecting the levels of Lactate in sweat. Electrolyte sensors measure the concentration of various electrolytes in blood or sweat; they mostly detect Chloride, Sodium and Potassium. Similarly, hydration sensors also detect the level of body hydration by measuring skin impedance or sweat composition.
- From the category of respiratory sensors, breath sensors use wearable patches or chest straps to measure the breathing rate and patterns. Capnography Sensors measure the efficiency of ventilation by measuring the concentration of carbon dioxide in exhaled air.
- From the neurological sensors category, Electroencephalogram (EEG) sensors record electrical activity of brain and, are often used in neurological monitoring and sleep study. Electromyography (EMG) sensors, on the other hand monitor muscle activity by detecting the electrical energy generated by muscle fibers.
- From the optical sensors category, Photoplethysmography (PPG) sensors measure changes in blood volume by using light; these are used for the applications of SPO_2 and heart rate monitoring. Spectroscopy sensors measure various physiological and biochemical properties by analyzing light absorption in tissues.
- There are various other sensors commonly used for the wearable applications: force sensors are used in posture monitoring and gait analysis as they could measure force exerted on a surface. Pressure sensors detect pressure changes and are used for detecting body position and respiratory functions. Humidity sensors can

detect the moisture level of human skin which could aid in the applications of comfort monitoring or hydration assessment.

- The above sensors may also be used in combination to achieve some advanced goal which might not be possible using a single sensor; a concept referred as multi-modal sensors. For example, health and activity monitoring could be done more efficiently by integrating gyroscope, accelerometer and heart rate sensor in a combined system.

Most of the wearable devices collect the required vital parameters continuously, however, they may also be configured to collect data at a pre-defined interval. In either case, the prevention and timely management of diseases become possible as compared to if the vitals are only monitored on the hospital visits. Therefore, continuous and remote health monitoring that is achieved by using wearable devices is one of the major driving forces behind the development of personalized medicine.

From the perspective of personalized medicine, the smart phones and wearable devices collect data that is being used for novel applications. For example, as discussed above, sleep tracking applications are being used in conjunction with smart watches to identify the sleep patterns; this information is then used for developing sleep-improving strategies and therapies for the patients. Previously, the patients had to stay at hospital facilities to get their sleep patterns studied, but now similar study has become possible from the comfort of patients' homes. Another common example is diabetes management, where the patients can use Bluetooth enabled glucose monitors or glucose monitoring patches to collect their glucose level information; this information can then be fed into simple IoT application, or into an advance AI based application, where predictions can be made for the next insulin dosage or diet plans. Even for the general population without having risk of any serious disease, the wearable devices may play a significant role by collecting data about their physical fitness and activity levels. This information is then used by the mobile apps and/or remote fitness experts to develop the customized exercise and diet plans. Hence, the wearable devices not only help to provide the customized diagnostics and diseases management opportunity, but also offer a tailored fitness management and disease prevention plan.

In addition to wearables that can be worn by the patients as a routine practice, there are also more advanced applications that require the patients to wear an IoT/AI enabled device while being physically present at a healthcare facility. One such example is the development of wearable device that measures ketone bodies [2], which play a crucial role in energy metabolism; these bodies are produced in the liver from fatty acids and various tissues/organs used them in the shortage of glucose. Particularly for diabetes patients, it is important to ensure that the level of ketone bodies remain satisfactory as their absence could affect the performance of brain/heart and other crucial organs. Therefore, electrochemical sensing platforms in the form of wearable devices have been developed to sense the presence of essential ketone bodies such as β-hydroxybutyrate (BHB).

Wearable chemical sensors have also been gaining popularity due to their potential of detecting biomarkers from human sweat, tears and saliva [3]. As compared to blood, the bio-fluid such as sweat is easier to acquire in order to measure proteins, hormones and metabolites. The mechanisms of field-effect transistor (FET), enzymatic recognition, frequency shift and ion-selective electrode (ISE) are often used for translating chemical information into electrical signals. The technologies mainly used for developing integrated wearable chemical sensors include flexible microfluidics and tattoo. Interestingly the chemical sensors can even be disposable, which offer an affordable and customizable solution for collecting data to be fed into personalized health systems. In addition to monitoring for bio-markers, wearable chemical sensors can also detect presence of pollutants in the environment.

Therapeutic Drug Monitoring (TDM) is another clinical practice where wearable sensing can offer guidance about the level of drugs available within the bloodstream of patients at fixed intervals [4]. The information about drug concentration is then used to adjust the subsequent drug dosages. Conventionally, TDM was done using chromatographic methods coupled with special detectors or immunoassays; however, these techniques suffered from the issues such as high instrumentation cost, lack of standardization and long turn-around time. Advancements in sensing and wearable technologies are expected to revolutionize this field of TDM by providing a quick and timely insight about the drug concentration in patient's bloodstream or other body fluids.

5.4.2 Smart Home Healthcare Solutions

Smart home offers a range of unique and customized services in addition to mere automation and control of home appliance. Ambient Assisted Living (AAL) is an emerging concept focused on providing independence to the elderly or physically challenged people living alone. AAL is supported mainly by wearables, biometric sensors, ambient environmental sensors, motion and activity sensors, telehealth platforms, mobile apps, smart home assistants/hubs, emergency response systems, and the technologies of IoT, AI, ML, big data analytics, cloud computing and Augmented and Virtual Reality (AR & VR). The core computing/communication technologies used by smart home, with a focus on healthcare service delivery are listed in Fig. 5.3: All these components come together for continuous health monitoring, chronic disease management and emergency alerts generation.

A typical smart home equipped with healthcare functionality is illustrated in Fig. 5.4. Fundamentally, a smart home collects data from wearable and implanted sensors as well as from ambient environmental sensors such as temperature, humidity and air quality. High-resolution webcams form an essential component of the home healthcare solutions as they not only monitor the presence of person in a certain location, but also detects situations such as fall; webcams integrated with advanced AI solutions can also detect the health conditions such as heart attacks or seizures. AI algorithms continuously analyze the footage received from smart home's webcams and detect abnormal postures, behaviors or movements such as facial twitching and rapid eye blinking which are often associated with seizures or

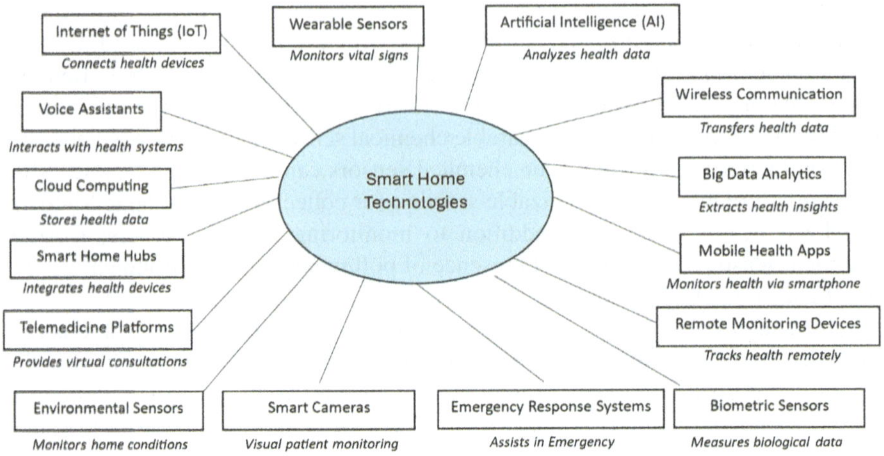

Fig. 5.3 Core technologies embedded with smart homes for healthcare

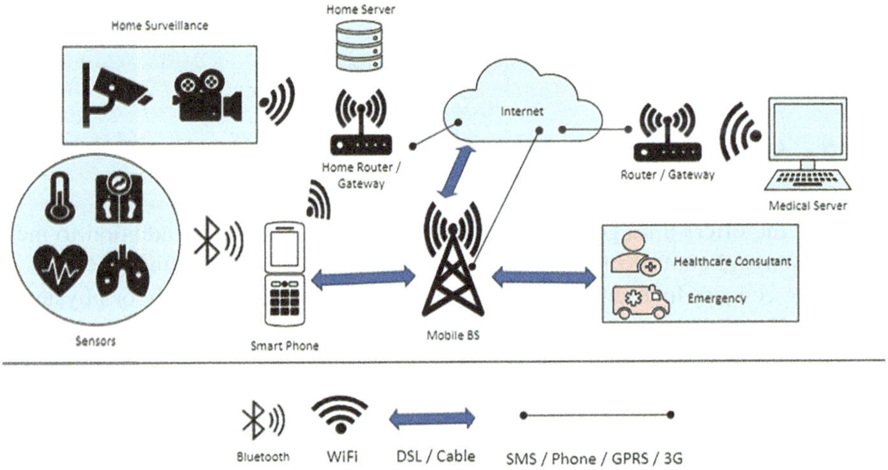

Fig. 5.4 Healthcare enabled smart home

heart attacks. ML models, furthermore, are trained on large seizures and cardiac diseases datasets to recognize the seizures which may occur in a smart home resident.

Digital Twins (DTs) are also being used to support the deployment of smart home as a healthcare solution. DT refers to a real-time physical replica of any physical object that is often used for simulation and analysis. DT is modeled as a smart home equipped with healthcare functionalities, focused on areas such as healthcare prediction, graphical monitoring and intelligent control [5]. The patients' vital data from the smart home can be simulated and fed into specialized ML algorithms for applications like fall detection, cardiovascular disease identification etc. As compared to other simulation systems, DT offers more varied datasets that reduce disparity between real-world and training data.

5.4.3 *Smartphone Based Immunosensors*

Conventionally, immunosensors have been known as solid-state biosensors that are used for measuring antibodies generated by certain bacteria. The major categories of immunosensors include electrochemical, microgravimetric and optical each used for detecting and quantifying specific antigens or antibodies in various samples with high sensitivity and specificity. Electrochemical immunosensors measure changes in electrical properties upon antigen-antibody binding, providing rapid and precise results. Microgravimetric immunosensors, such as quartz crystal microbalance (QCM) sensors, detect mass changes on a sensor surface due to antigen-antibody interactions, making them useful for real-time monitoring of binding events. Optical immunosensors, including surface plasmon resonance (SPR) and fluorescence-based sensors, rely on changes in light properties, such as intensity or wavelength, upon antigen-antibody binding, offering highly sensitive and label-free detection methods.

With the increasing advancements and application scope of smartphones, smartphone based immunosensors have been developed. These have been used for collecting samples for quick on-site screening of various bio-markers in an efficient and cost-effective way [6]. As smartphones are used by majority of the global population today, their use for clinical purposes offers a semi-automated method that can serve with a minimal intervention; users can perform common diagnostic tests from the comfort of their homes, which further enhances the scope of remote monitoring (which was earlier relying on data collected merely from the wearable sensors). For example, a smartphone-based device using advanced methods of magnetoelastic immuno-sensing has been developed to measure *C*-Reaction protein (CRP), which is a marker of nonspecific immunity for vital signs and wound assessment [7]. Conventionally, measuring CRP has been a complex process which required hospital-based instruments and high-cost reagents; now, the smartphone can be combined with system-on-chip (SoC) hardware architecture for performing the same test.

5.4.4 *Artificial Intelligence for Cancer Medication*

Advancements in AI and their integration with smart health systems have enhanced the diagnostic accuracy and drug development efficiency. AI speeds up the processes of customized vaccine and medication development for patients based on their continuous monitoring and genetic analysis. Particularly for cancer, personalized medicine appears as a game changer as AI algorithms offers a considerable opportunity for early detection and customized therapies for targeting specific genetic mutations. Today, various AI techniques are being used for diagnosing, treating cancers; some of them are listed in Table 5.1:

The major motivation for using AI for cancer medication is highly heterogenous effects of surgical methods or drugs used in patients; the patients with same tumor may have different curative effects after undergoing similar treatment. Therefore, there is a crucial need of assessing the impact of medication on tumors of specific patients, such as changes in their proteins, genes and cancer cell phenotypes. With the help of AI and big data, it becomes possible to identify the hidden patterns in enormous amount of data. For example, detailed insights about digital pathological images, radiomics, proteomics, transcriptomics and genomics can be mined using machine and deep learning algorithms [8]. Moreover, new biomarkers can also be identified from the bulky data for assisting the processes of tumor screening, detection, diagnosis, treatment as well as prediction of prognosis.

5.4.5 Healthcare Recommender Systems (HRSs)

HRSs are specialized information systems designed to assist patients, healthcare providers, and other stakeholders in making informed health-related decisions. These systems use technologies of AI, ML and data analytics to identify the health patterns of users and make the required recommendations about medication dosages, diet plans, exercise routines, diagnostic tests, physician appointments etc. A typical recommender system learns from the user behavior and past health history and recommends the best options with a goal of optimizing the patient outcomes. The use of advanced AI algorithms improves the prediction and hence, the recommendation accuracy; the AI techniques used for healthcare recommender system include deep neural networks, active learning, transfer learning, reinforcement learning and fuzzy logic and rules.

Despite having numerous advantages of deploying AI algorithms for personalized recommender systems, there are also some challenges that incur while using them. First, data sparsity often arises due to the users only providing feedback about limited items; this could result in the recommender system offering unreasonable recommendations to the users who had not provided any feedback [9]. The issue of data sparsity can be solved by relying on the social connections of users and drawing inferences from the feedback provided by them. Second, diversity may occur if the recommender system tends to recommend the items which are either way too similar to the users' preferences or are very different from them. Clearly, in both of these situations, the recommender system might leave some systems which it would have recommended in case it had not considered the user preferences. The technique of linear time closed itemset miner (LCM) is used to increase the diversity of recommender system by identifying the frequent item sets. Third major challenge is known as cold start: it often happens with both new or existing users, when the system does not find enough metadata. For example, when a new user joins and the

Table 5.1 Key AI algorithms used for cancer diagnosis and treatment

S. no.	AI algorithm	Purpose
1	Convolutional Neural Networks (CNNs)	Image analysis for cancer detection in medical imaging.
2	Support Vector Machines (SVMs)	Classification of cancer types based on biomarkers.
3	Random Forest	Feature selection and prediction of cancer outcomes.
4	Deep Learning	Complex data analysis for personalized cancer treatment.
5	Natural Language Processing (NLP)	Analysis of clinical notes and research data for cancer research and treatment.
6	Artificial Neural Networks (ANNs)	Pattern recognition and data mining in cancer research.
7	K-nearest neighbors (KNN)	Classification of cancer types based on similarity to known cases.
8	Decision Trees	Interpretation of complex datasets to guide cancer treatment decisions.
9	Genetic Algorithms	Optimization of cancer treatment plans based on genetic data.
10	Bayesian Networks	Probabilistic modeling of cancer risk factors and treatment outcomes.
11	Gradient Boosting Machines (GBM)	Ensemble learning for predicting cancer prognosis and treatment response.
12	Long Short-Term Memory (LSTM)	Deep learning model for analyzing sequential medical data in cancer progression.
13	Principal Component Analysis (PCA)	Dimensionality reduction technique to identify key features and patterns in cancer datasets.
14	Fuzzy Logic	Handling uncertainty in medical data for cancer diagnosis and treatment decision-making.
15	Clustering Algorithms (e.g., K-means)	Grouping similar patient profiles to personalize cancer treatment plans.
16	Markov Models	Analyzing sequential data to predict cancer progression and outcomes.
17	Ensemble Learning (e.g., AdaBoost)	Combining multiple algorithms to improve accuracy in cancer classification and prediction tasks.
18	Deep Belief Networks	Unsupervised learning for feature extraction and representation in cancer research.
19	Reinforcement Learning	Optimizing treatment strategies over time based on patient responses and outcomes.
20	Autoencoders	Unsupervised learning for dimensionality reduction and feature extraction in cancer genomics and imaging data.
21	Logistic Regression	Modeling the probability of cancer occurrence based on risk factors.
22	Naive Bayes	Probability-based classification for cancer subtype prediction.
23	Survival Analysis	Modeling time-to-event outcomes in cancer prognosis and treatment planning.

(continued)

Table 5.1 (continued)

S. no.	AI algorithm	Purpose
24	Hidden Markov Models (HMMs)	Analyzing temporal patterns in cancer progression and treatment response.
25	Gaussian Processes	Bayesian approach for modeling uncertainty and predicting cancer outcomes based on prior data.
26	Radial Basis Function Networks (RBFNs)	Non-linear data modeling for cancer diagnosis based on features.
27	Metaheuristic Algorithms	Optimization techniques for personalized cancer treatment planning based on patient-specific data.
28	Swarm Intelligence Algorithms	Mimicking natural swarm behavior to optimize cancer treatment strategies.
29	Anomaly Detection Algorithms	Identifying unusual patterns in cancer data that may indicate novel or rare cases requiring specialized treatment approaches.
30	Recurrent Neural Networks (RNNs)	Analyzing sequential data such as time-series patient data for cancer progression monitoring.
31	Transfer Learning	Utilizing pre-trained models to adapt knowledge from one cancer type to another with limited data.
32	Multi-task Learning	Simultaneously learning multiple related tasks in cancer research and treatment, enhancing prediction accuracy.
33	Graph Neural Networks	Analyzing relationships and interactions between genes or proteins in cancer molecular networks.
34	Deep Reinforcement Learning	Optimizing cancer treatment plans dynamically based on patient responses and clinical outcomes over time.
35	Self-organizing Maps (SOMs)	Unsupervised learning for clustering and visualizing complex cancer datasets.
36	Bayesian Optimization	Efficiently optimizing hyperparameters in machine learning models used for cancer prediction and treatment.
37	Elastic Net	Combining L1 and L2 regularization techniques for feature selection in cancer genomics and biomarker identification.
38	Manifold Learning	Dimensionality reduction techniques for visualizing high-dimensional cancer data in lower-dimensional spaces.
39	Ordinal Regression	Predicting ordinal outcomes in cancer prognosis, such as stages or grades, based on patient data and biomarkers.

recommender system does not have any user preference data to offer recommendations, the cold start problem arises. Naïve Bayes techniques are usually implemented to deal with the cold start where items can be estimated without having the previous history. Finally, scalability has also become a challenge with the modern recommender systems as they are expected to process lots of data and generate quick recommendations. One-dimensionality reduction techniques are used to deal with scalability by eliminating data sparsity and dividing data into smaller chunks for quick processing.

5.4.6 Quantum Computing for Sequencing Bioinformatics

Quantum computing is the futuristic technology which is also expected to play a major role in personalized medicine due to its capability of examining geonomics data at a very high speed. Although Bioinformatics technology has matured enough to apply computational tools for analyzing the biological data, these tools often lack capacity to deal with the complexity and volume of biological data. Therefore, when AI and cloud computing will be combined with quantum computing, it would become possible to develop highly scalable health solutions focused on sequencing (a process to determine the order of nucleotides in DNA or RNA) [10]. First, quantum computing would allow solving complex problems involving large datasets and algorithms; secondly, most of the tasks related to genome sequencing such as genome assembly, alignment, and motif finding requires optimization, which is a key feature of quantum computing; for example, the algorithms Grover's and Shor's would significantly increase the processing speed [11].

When used in sequencing, quantum computing can support various applications. It could optimize the process of genome assembly, where short reads are assembled into complete genomes. The time required for this process with traditional computing is in months and days, which could be reduced to hours through quantum computing methods. Similarly, another critical task in bioinformatics is aligning sequences to reference genomes; quantum computation can also offer more efficient and faster alignment algorithms. Quantum computing can also influence the area of protein folding, which requires the understanding of how proteins fold based on sequence data; accurate predicting the protein folding can lead to advances in drug discovery and development. Furthermore, quantum computing could also enhance the complex statistical models required for Identifying genetic variants from sequencing data; this could lead to Identifying genetic variants from sequencing data.

5.4.7 Gene Sequencing and Editing

Next-Generation Sequencing (NGS) technologies have been used for analyzing genomes of patients. Various genetic variations and mutations can be identified through NGS, such as SNPs and CNVs. Genome-Wide Association Studies (GWAS) is another technique that has been used for identifying associations between genetic variations and specific diseases by scanning the genomes of multiple patients, generating large datasets; it helps to identify the genetic factors contributing to the risk of each disease and response to each drug. Moreover, another gene-editing technology commonly used is CRISPR-Cas9 that can correct the genetic mutations at their source.

5.5 Ethical Challenges

Deploying the cutting-edge computing technologies for personalized medicine create many ethical challenges. The efficiency of data analytics and AI techniques totally depends on the availability of data; lack of data quality or availability for specific population sector may result in inaccurate analysis or recommendations, even for the personalized systems. In addition to data, it is also a crucial task to select the best machine learning algorithm for each healthcare problem; unlike other domains, the choice of algorithm would be of utmost importance for the healthcare sector, as it could risk the entire diagnostic and treatment plan. The diversity of health-related problems also creates challenges for the selection of best algorithm; here, it is to be noted that the algorithm that works well for one patient may not offer an optimal performance for another patient with a similar disease; as previously discussed, this mainly happens due to the unique genetic make-up and other characteristics of patients.

Similarly, there is an associated lack of evidence and reproducibility for every machine learning model which could also affect the efficiency of healthcare systems relying on these technologies. There are also issues related to the lack of understanding for AI model process and prediction; the computer scientists and medical practitioners need to work in close collaboration for the sake of efficient development/implementation of AI algorithm for a specific healthcare problem. Moreover, developing the accountability framework/guidelines regarding the deployment and continued use of computing systems in the domain of personalized systems is also a challenge.

The increased reliance on the computing systems and devices (such as wearables) is expected to significantly impact the physician-patient relationship and interaction, which may reduce the human-level emotional understanding and empathy during the treatment/therapy process. Moreover, there are major privacy challenges associated with the creation, sharing and distribution of patient data. There are various possibilities when it comes to access and rights over patient data; for example, the users not actually authorized might have access to patient data, whereas the stakeholders which should actually be given access may only have a partial access. Clearly, for personalized medicine, there is a lot of data to be shared including patients' family and medical history and the issues such as data ownership and patient consent for data sharing or analysis have not yet been fully addressed; the privacy concerns, therefore, make one of the major reasons why these technologies are not largely adopted despite having a proven socio-economic and health benefit.

References

1. S. Hornstein, K. Zantvoort, U. Lueken, B. Funk, K. Hilbert, Personalization strategies in digital mental health interventions: A systematic review and conceptual framework for depressive symptoms. Front. Digit. Health **5** (2023). https://doi.org/10.3389/fdgth.2023.1170002

2. R. Del Caño, T. Saha, C. Moonla, E. De la Paz, J. Wang, Ketone bodies detection: Wearable and mobile sensors for personalized medicine and nutrition. TrAC Trends Anal. Chem. **159** (2023). https://doi.org/10.1016/j.trac.2023.116938
3. T. He, F. Wen, Y. Yang, X. Le, W. Liu, C. Lee, Emerging wearable chemical sensors enabling advanced integrated systems toward personalized and preventive medicine. Anal. Chem. **95**(1) (2023). https://doi.org/10.1021/acs.analchem.2c04527
4. H.C. Ates, J.A. Roberts, J. Lipman, A.E.G. Cass, G.A. Urban, C. Dincer, On-site therapeutic drug monitoring. Trends Biotechnol. **38**(11) (2020). https://doi.org/10.1016/j.tibtech.2020.03.001
5. J. Chen et al., Digital twin empowered wireless healthcare monitoring for smart home. IEEE J. Sel. Areas Commun. **41**(11) (2023). https://doi.org/10.1109/JSAC.2023.3310097
6. H. Kholafazad-Kordasht, M. Hasanzadeh, F. Seidi, Smartphone based immunosensors as next generation of healthcare tools: Technical and analytical overview towards improvement of personalized medicine. TrAC Trends Anal. Chem. **145** (2021). https://doi.org/10.1016/j.trac.2021.116455
7. Z. Yuan et al., A cost-effective smartphone-based device for rapid C-reaction protein (CRP) detection using magnetoelastic immunosensor. Lab Chip **23**(8) (2023). https://doi.org/10.1039/d2lc01065h
8. J. Liao et al., Artificial intelligence assists precision medicine in cancer treatment. Front. Oncol. **12** (2023). https://doi.org/10.3389/fonc.2022.998222
9. T. Iqbal et al., Towards integration of artificial intelligence into medical devices as a real-time recommender system for personalised healthcare: State-of-the-art and future prospects. Health Sci. Rev. **10** (2024). https://doi.org/10.1016/j.hsr.2024.100150
10. S. Goswami, S. Sharma, Artificial intelligence, quantum computing and cloud computing enabled personalized medicine in next generation sequencing bioinformatics, in *2024 IEEE International Conference on Interdisciplinary Approaches in Technology and Management for Social Innovation, IATMSI 2024*, (2024). https://doi.org/10.1109/IATMSI60426.2024.10502533
11. J. Davids, N. Lidströmer, H. Ashrafian, Artificial intelligence in medicine using quantum computing in the future of healthcare. Artif. Intell. Med. (2022). https://doi.org/10.1007/978-3-030-64573-1_338

Chapter 6
Revolutionizing Digital Imaging

6.1 Evolution of Digital Imaging

Medical imaging is a means of visualizing the interior of a body for clinical analysis and medical intervention. Many imaging modalities were developed by the start of the digital era, all with different strengths and weaknesses [1]. Plain film radiography represented an inexpensive and available first-line technique useful in trauma and joint diseases where high spatial resolution exists, but it had poor soft-tissue contrast. Fluoroscopy, the first ionizing radiation technique, enabled live imaging useful for diagnostic and procedural work but involved a large amount of radiation exposure and poor soft tissue detail. Computed Tomography (CT) provided detailed cross-sectional images and was relatively inexpensive but required high dosages of radiation, had poor spatial resolution, and was time-consuming. Nuclear medicine provided important functional information using radioactive material but involved radiation exposure, patient preparation, and poor spatial resolution. Though Magnetic Resonance Imaging [MRI] held an unbeatable position regarding soft tissue contrast without ionizing radiation, it was time-consuming, less available, and it required patient cooperation. Angiography provided highly detailed vascular images but was invasive, with risks from contrast agents in the procedure. Interventional radiology reduced surgical risks and costs by imaging guidance for procedures but required specialized equipment and expertise [2].

Modern digital imaging techniques have contributed much to completely revolutionize medical imaging for more accurate diagnosis and planning of treatment. Some key advances include digital X-ray detectors, such as flat panel detectors, considerably improved the image quality with a reduced radiation exposure in comparison to film-screen radiography. Advances in computed tomography scanners achieved higher resolution images acquired within faster times and with a lower radiation dose. Improvements in magnet strength, gradient performance, and the

S. Siddiqui et al., *Connected Health Insights for Sustainable Development*,
https://doi.org/10.1007/978-3-031-81433-4_6

design of pulse sequences have improved the quality of MRI images, enabling better tissue contrast to be obtained with faster scanning. In ultrasound imaging, digital beamforming and improved transducer technology have yielded higher-resolution images with better tissue penetration. Specifically, digital mammography has benefited from the introduction of full-field digital mammography systems that provide better contrast, image quality, and reduced radiation exposure compared to screen-film mammography. The advances in these digital imaging modalities have therefore enabled the development of computer-aided detection systems, which would aid radiologists in the detection and diagnosis of diseases. Digital images can also be stored, retrieved, and transmitted easily to enable telemedicine and remote diagnosis [3, 4].

Moreover, growth in computational powers has brought in its wake burgeoning image processing algorithms. Machine Learning (ML), Deep Learning (DL), and data science are major drivers of this revolution as they have stormed the field of medical imaging. Accurate interpretation through ML and DL algorithms of a myriad of medical pictures aids timely diagnosis, thus personalized disease-tailored treatment, for improved patient outcome. At the same time, data science uses these huge volumes of data produced as by-products from medical imaging to display deep insights into trends in diseases, treatment outcomes, and patient results [5].

6.2 Role of Machine and Deep Learning in Digital Imaging

The advent of ML and DL has revolutionized the field of digital imaging. These technologies have enabled unprecedented advancements in various applications, including image classification, segmentation, object detection, in medical imaging. This chapter explores the fundamental principles and major contributions of ML and DL techniques in digital imaging, emphasizing key architectures, methodologies, and their practical implications.

6.2.1 Convolutional Neural Networks (CNNs)

Convolutional Neural Networks (CNNs) [6], are the cornerstone of many deep learning applications in digital imaging. Their design inherently enables automatic and adaptive learning of spatial hierarchies of features from the input images, so they are very suitable for image classification, segmentation, and object detection tasks. The taxonomy for a better understanding is presented in Fig. 6.1.

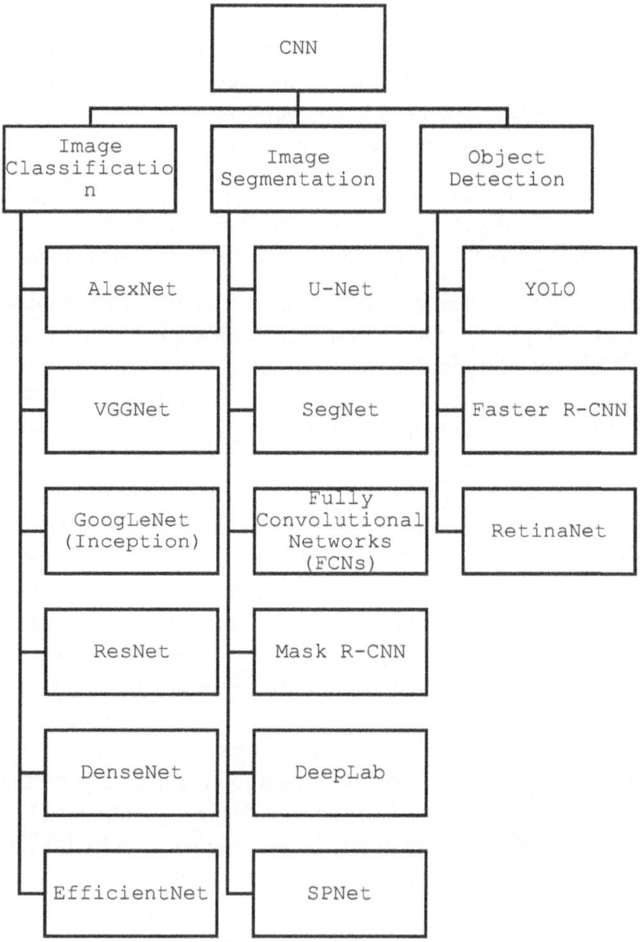

Fig. 6.1 Taxonomy of CNN models used in digital imaging

6.2.2 Image Classification

Image classification involves categorizing images into predefined classes [7]. Several CNN architectures have been pivotal in advancing image classification:

- AlexNet
- AlexNet [8], was a groundbreaking model that won the ImageNet Large Scale Visual Recognition Challenge (ILSVRC). There are eight layers in the model: five convolutional layers and three fully connected layers. Major innovations taken out from the AlexNet model are concerned with ReLU activation for adding non-linearity, dropout to avoid overfitting, and efficient use of GPUs during the training of large datasets.

- Trained for large datasets of medical images, AlexNet can tell the presence of cancerous tissues represented on mammograms, MRI scans, and histopathology slides. Convolutional layers will help AlexNet retrieve features distinguishing normal from abnormal tissues, all of which can contribute to early cancer diagnosis, for example, breast, lung, and skin cancer.
- Subsequently, AlexNet has been applied to detecting diabetic retinopathy and age-related macular degeneration from retinal images. It supports timely diagnosis and treatment by recognizing subtle changes in retinal structures.
- Furthermore, AlexNet can classify various organs/tissues from CT and MRI scans, thereby helping in the automated radiological image interpretation process. It has also been trained to classify diseases from chest X-rays, identifying conditions such as pneumonia, tuberculosis, and lately, COVID-19, thereby helping radiologists to prioritize cases.
- VGGNet
- VGGNet [9], proposed by the Visual Geometry Group at the University of Oxford, is known for its simplicity and depth. The most noted version would be VGG-16, which has 13 convolutional layers and 3 fully connected layers. VGGNet uses small 3 × 3 filters and max-pooling layers with consistency, which is an excellent balance between depth and computational efficiency. With the deep architecture of VGGNet, it can extract intrinsic features from medical images; therefore, disease classification using these images goes very well with this approach.
- VGGNet can classify histopathology images to help distinguish between benign and malignant tumors. It is deep, allowing it to note lines of very fine differences in tissue structure indicative of cancer. VGGNet also evaluates chest X-rays and CT scans for illnesses like pneumonia, tuberculosis, and COVID-19. With its high accuracy, it supports radiologists in early diagnosis.
- GoogLeNet (Inception)
- Fang et al. proposed GoogLeNet [10] also known as an Inception network, which majorly differs in the use of Inception modules. This module makes it use multiple convolution filters in parallel to capture different levels of abstraction. Use of 1 × 1 convolutions reduces dimensionality, hence computational cost, therefore is economical. This also gives the needed flexibility to GoogLeNet in medical imaging, where the potential ability to capture multiscale features becomes highly significant.
- The Inception modules strongly empower GoogLeNet, enabling the extraction of features in one pass at multiple scales. This is a very useful characteristic of medical imaging, since different structures, such as tumors or even organs like the brain, liver, and lungs, are basically of different sizes and shapes. It makes the network recognize tumors of various sizes and shapes within the medical images like MRI and CT scans. It is able to process at different scales, making GoogLeNet more effective at lesion identification and analysis within the dermatological images, hence more accurate at diagnosing conditions relating to the skin.

- Low computational load makes GoogLeNet feasible for deployment in clinical settings where fast processing times are a requirement for real-time diagnostics. Deep architecture and the use of Inception modules utilize the high accuracy and robustness of GoogLeNet in distinguishing different diseases, such as types of cancers or lung conditions, from X-rays and CT scans. The model supports automated interpretation and diagnosis by accurately classifying different organs and tissues from radiological images.
- ResNet
- Residual Networks, or ResNet [11]. This architecture makes it possible to train deep networks due to residual blocks with skip connections that help maintain gradient flow during backpropagation, hence much deeper—ResNet-50, ResNet-101—without causing degradation. The implementation has specific advantages for medical image classification.
- The main innovation of ResNet was that it linked residual learning with the concept of shortcut connections, which enabled it to train much more depth without suffering the vanishing gradient problem. Since deeper networks can extract more complex or abstract features from medical images, this will lead to more accurate classification. For instance, in the case of histopathological image analysis, deeper layers can capture very small variations in cellular structure indicative of different cancers. By residual connections, deeper architectures are less prone to overfitting, a primordial consideration in most medical imaging applications where the amount of labeled data may be scarce.
- ResNet applies to multi-class classification problems within medical imaging, specifically the identification of different types of pneumonia, lung cancer stages, and brain tumor types from a CT or MRI scan. Most of the medical images are noisy and contain several artifacts. Residual connections add depth to ResNet and enable the model to emphasize relevant features and reduce false positives, thereby being more robust.
- Medical image tasks can be performed using variants of ResNets tailored to different applications, such as ResNet-50 and ResNet-101. In this way, balance between computational efficiency and performance can be attained. It can be combined with other models like U-Net for segmentation, further enhancing results for tasks which require both classification and localization of medical features.
- DenseNet
- DenseNet stands for Densely Connected Convolutional Networks [12], connects every layer to all other layers through feed-forward. The dense connectivity does not lose any information during forward diffusion from one layer to another; on the contrary, it enhances feature reusage, reducing the total number of parameters required compared to traditional networks. This unique approach provides several advantages for medical imaging tasks.
- DenseNet connects each layer to every other layer in a feed-forward way: each layer takes all of the feature maps computed up to that point as input. This architecture makes sure that the features computed in the early layers are directly available to all the later layers during feature learning. Similar to ResNet,

DenseNet avoids the vanishing gradient problem but does so by maximizing information flow between layers, thus being enormously successful in training very deep networks.

- It has more parameter efficiency due to the dense connections within this network. By encouraging feature reuse, DenseNet achieves comparable or better performance with fewer parameters than other deep networks, which is very vital in medical imaging, where computational resources can sometimes be limited.
- DenseNet does well on fine-grained image classification tasks, such as the different stages of diseases picked out from imaging data and the stages of diabetic retinopathy from retinal images. Spatial feature learning is further enhanced by dense connections, which are advantageously applied in segmentation tasks like delineating tumors in MRI or segmenting organs in CT scans.
- EfficientNet

- EfficientNet [13], employs compound scaling to balance network depth, width, and resolution. This balances the scaling approach with the highly efficient architecture of EfficientNet, which is particularly useful for tasks in medical imaging. It attains high accuracy with fewer parameters, hence appropriate for mobile and edge devices. This method is pushing forward new state-of-the-art benchmarks on image classification tasks based on performance and efficiency.

- EfficientNet scales depth, width, and resolution uniformly by using a compound coefficient, which is the design obtained by balancing the three magic variables through the technique of compound scaling. This ensures a proper use of the parameters and computational resources instead of relatively arbitrary scaling of architectures. The balanced approach thus leads to state-of-the-art performance in a list of various image classification benchmarks, which does channel to the medical imaging domain with high accuracy.

- EfficientNet has been proven to be more accurate in image classification, which is a big deal in medical applications, where the smallest detail can affect the life of a patient. And researchers/developers can select different model scales (e.g., EfficientNet-B0 to EfficientNet-B7) according to the specific requirements of medical imaging while reaching a good trade-off between speed and accuracy. The efficient architecture of this model enables it to be deployed in edge devices, under such a setup that makes it feasible to be used in point-of-care settings or very remote locations.

6.2.3 Image Segmentation

Image segmentation divides an image into meaningful segments, often used to identify objects or regions of interest. Accurate segmentation of medical images is essential for tasks such as identifying tumor boundaries, delineating anatomical structures, and guiding surgical procedures [14]. This section explores how advanced deep learning models, specifically U-Net, SegNet, Fully Convolutional Networks (FCNs), Mask R-CNN, DeepLab, and PSPNet (Pyramid Scene Parsing Network), contribute to the field of medical image segmentation.

- U-Net

- U-Net [15] is widely used in biomedical image segmentation by using an encoder-decoder architecture along with skip connections that merge the high-resolution features of the encoder with up sampled features of the decoder for location accuracy. It excels in tasks where exact localization is required, such as the segmentation of tumors from MRI, extraction of organs from CT images, and cell boundaries from microscopy images. Skip connections between encoder and decoder conserve spatial information and hence deliver accurate segmentations. U-Net works very well on a limited amount of annotated training data, which happens to be quite common in medical imaging.
- SegNet
- SegNet [16] which is an encoder-decoder network for pixel-wise image segmentation. The encoder is what makes up the convolutional layers, while the decoder utilizes corresponding pooling indices from the encoder before up sampling the same. Thus, SegNet remains very useful for real-time applications such as intra-operative image analysis and segmentation of large datasets like whole-slide histopathology images. Using pooling indices can reduce the number of parameters and, more importantly, the computational cost; hence SegNet is very suitable for real-time processing. It is also good at handling changes in input data, a very important point in medical imaging where the quality of imagery may be very different from one image to another.
- Fully Convolutional Networks (FCNs)
- FCNs [17] replace fully connected layers with convolutional layers, which makes the network capable of processing images of any size and returning a segmentation map. They are able to capture spatial hierarchies efficiently and turn out to be very basics in many segmentation tasks. They have applications for organ segmentation of CT and MRI scans, detection of brain lesions, and segmentation of retinal vessels in fundus images. FCNs enable end-to-end trainability and inference, greatly simplifying the segmentation pipeline. FCNs can exploit and generalize quite a good number of medical imaging tasks by incorporating domain-specific modifications.
- Mask R-CNN
- Mask R-CNN [18] are extensions of Faster R-CNN that append another branch to predict segmentation masks on each RoI. In view of this, the architecture is very outstanding for tasks related to object detection and segmentation. Mask R-CNN is especially good in situations where instance segmentation should be done as different instances include the case of individual cells in microscopy images or segmenting multiple tumors in radiology scans and sometimes even segmenting/delineating overlapping anatomical structures. Especially in applications where differentiation among individual objects is most needed, the instance segmentation ability gives it high value. Mask R-CNN provides fine details of segmentation masks, thereby increasing the accuracy in medical image analysis.

- DeepLab
- DeepLab [19], uses atrous (or dilated) convolutions to encode multiscale context and Conditional Random Fields for accurate delineation of boundaries. Further variants, such as DeepLabv3+, still improve the accuracy in segmentation. DeepLab has applications for segmenting complex structures from medical images, like the brain tissues from MRI, lung fields in chest X-rays, and pathological regions from histopathology images. Thus, atrous convolutions combined with ASPP allow DeepLab to encode fine details and broader contextual information. The architecture of DeepLab is flexibly adaptable to many segmentation tasks, making it a flexible tool within medical imaging.
- SPNet (Pyramid Scene Parsing Network)

- PSPNet [20] uses a pyramid pooling module that recovered the global context information in different scales, improving the segmentation of scenes that have complex structures. PSPNet can be used for segmentation of large anatomical structures and modeling of spatial relations between different regions in medical images, like whole-body MRI segmentation and delineation of organs in CT images. Another key component of PSPNet is the pyramid pooling module, which allows the network to capture local and global context and, therefore, help to improve the segmentation accuracy in complex scenes. It has leading performance on various segmentation benchmarks, making it a reliable choice for medical image segmentation tasks.

6.2.4 Object Detection

Object detection in medical imaging is a critical task for the identification and localization of regions of interest within medical images such as X-rays, CT scans, and MRIs. Diagnosis of diseases, planning of treatments, and follow-up on progress rely on this process. Traditional methods almost always rest on manual inspection by radiologists, which can be time-consuming and prone to human error. Object detection systems have been enabled to be quite effective with advances in machine learning, more specifically Convolutional Neural Networks or CNNs. Such systems permit quick and highly accurate detection of abnormalities like tumors, lesions, and fractures, hence greatly improving diagnostic efficiency and accuracy. State-of-the-art detection models with large datasets and sophisticated algorithms, like YOLO, Faster R-CNN, and RetinaNet, will engulf the associated complexity and variability of medical imaging, hence forming robust tools to help bring better patient outcomes and support a physician in his or her decision-making.

- YOLO (You Only Look Once)

- YOLO [21], is a real-time object detection system reassembling the object detection as a single regression problem, straight from full image pixels to bounding box coordinates and class probabilities. This paper divides an entire input image into a grid and predicts bounding boxes and probabilities for each grid cell. Due to this unified model architecture in YOLO, it enables the framework to be very fast in comparison to traditional approaches of object detection, which involve several stages of processing.

- YOLO processes images in real-time and achieves high frames per second rates. Hence, it can be applied in all those areas where decisions have to be made in a very short span of time. Although fast, YOLO exhibits impressive accuracy in applications for object detection tasks. In its design, there are very minimal background errors. It correctly identifies the objects in the images. The unified architecture makes the training process easy to implement and fine-tune.

- YOLO identifies and localizes bones, fractures, and other important anatomical features from an X-ray image quickly and with great accuracy. Badging YOLO into noisy, varied data, it can be applied to the detection and classification of varied structures like organs, tumors, and other abnormalities in CT imaging, thus offering rapid diagnostic support. In YOLO, the speed and accuracy help in detecting lesions, tumors, or any other abnormal tissue regions using MRI scans. It helps quickly interpret vast amounts of imaging data.
- Faster R-CNN
- Faster R-CNN [22], is a more advanced object detection model based on an integrated framework of Fast R-CNN and an 'in-house' Region Proposal Network. The latter generates region proposals, which are used by the detection network to further refine such proposals and classify objects. This kind of integration makes it possible for Fast R-CNN to improve in efficiency and accuracy in detecting objects, due to the streamlining of the process for generating region proposals and object classification.
- Faster R-CNN is known for its capability to detect with high accuracy, thus offering this accuracy in object identification and localization within images. It generates region proposals efficiently via the RPN, which reduces computational cost compared to traditional methods.: It can process different scales of objects within an image, thus very versatile for a number of medical image analysis tasks.
- Faster R-CNN methods can identify microcalcification, masses, and other indicators of breast cancer from a mammogram image with high accuracy. Hence, it helps in the earlier diagnosis of this disease. This method has done admirably well at the tasks of identification of abnormalities like nodules, tumors, and organ irregularities from CT images with accurate localization and classification. Faster R-CNN applied in MRI imaging can cover a wide variety of recognition and classification, including brain structures, lesions, and other anomalies, hence helping neurological assessment and formulation of a treatment plan.
- RetinaNet

- RetinaNet [23] is the state-of-the-art object detection, which fundamentally improves class imbalance through the uses of a focal loss function. Integrating the Feature Pyramid Network into the model, then, is a better and more efficient scheme for detecting objects at multiple scales and improving accuracy on small objects and densely packed scenes. The focal loss function raises weights on hard examples, making a model do better in imbalanced datasets.

- RetinaNet architecture with a focal loss function empowers this model to detect small and densely packed objects easily missed by other models. Applying FPN on RetinaNet Making use of features at all scales for improving accuracy in detecting objects at different sizes. Certainly, RetinaNet works best in identifying small lesions within medical images, as tiny tumors or even microaneurysms are always terribly critical for diagnostic processes and consequent treatment. It will work well for the detection and classification of small abnormalities on X-ray images, such as small fractures, nodules, and other vital findings often missed by less sensitive models. This places RetinaNet in a very special position due to its inherent class imbalance property and small object detection ability, making it more appropriate for the identification of subtle anomalies in CT and MRI scans.

6.3 Recurrent Neural Networks (RNNs)

RNNs [24] tend to play a big role in medical imaging, with most tasks involving sequential data and time series analysis. Most medical imaging data comes in sequences: video frames in ultrasound imaging, slices in MRI or CT scans, and time series data in echocardiograms. RNNs, especially their variants—Long Short-Term Memory and Gated Recurrent Units—are particularly tailor-made for analyzing such sequential data. The paper discusses current applications of RNNs in medical imaging, alluding to how they help advancement in the area.

One class of neural networks whose functionality is majorly associated with sequential data is recurrent neural networks. Each representational unit of information—a hidden state—is maintained internally to capture information about all past elements in the sequence. In basic RNNs, at every time step, the hidden state gets updated by the current input and the prior hidden state. The information may be extracted from the hidden state to study a forecast or passed on to the next time step. Taxonomy of RNNs is presented in Fig. 6.2.

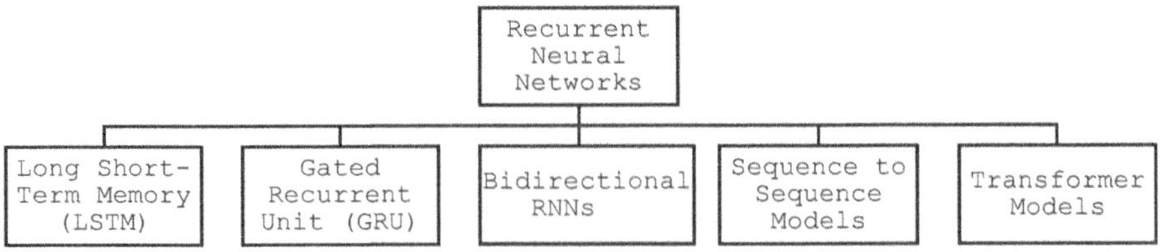

Fig. 6.2 Taxonomy of RNN models used in digital imaging

6.3.1 Long Short-Term Memory (LSTM)

Basically, Long Short-Term Memory [25] networks are a class of RNNs specifically designed to help the basic RNN overcome the limitations involved in very long-term dependencies. LSTMs do this with memory cells and three major gates: an input gate, a forget gate, and an output gate. Those gates control the flow of information in such a way that the LSTM is able to maintain and update information of the cell state over these long sequences.

The most useful areas of application for LSTMs in medical imaging involve image sequences, such as slices in an MRI or CT scan. By doing so, they manage to capture long-range dependencies and temporal patterns that are crucial for disease advancement identification and context comprehension in a series of images. For instance, using a series of MRI scans, LSTMs can be used to track changes in tumor size over time, helping in assessing the effectiveness of treatment. Furthermore, LSTMs can generate medical reports while processing sequences of image features in a coherent and contextually accurate description.

These are recurrent neural networks that have been developed to be able to finally capture long-term dependencies in sequential data. This structure consists of an encoder and a decoder. The encoder processes the input sequence and encodes it into a context vector. The decoder then makes use of this context vector for output generation at every subsequent step.

In medical imaging, LSTM-based models find a fine description of medical reports based on sequences of images. LSTM-based models go through image feature sequences, which are extracted from modalities like MRIs, CT scans, or ultrasounds, to bear the logic of how a medical condition evolves over time. The LSTMs can generate coherent and contextually relevant text reports owing to the encoding of the sequence of observations. For instance, the sequential growth of a tumor in MRI images or summary of findings from a series of ultrasound frames. This model helps in bringing out consistency in the reports because the dependencies are kept along the time axis. The logic of the LSTM model ensures accurate and appropriate descriptions of medical conditions.

6.3.2 Gated Recurrent Unit (GRU)

GRUs [26], are a simplification of an LSTM. There is an update gate in the input and forget gates, cutting down parameters, thus leading to a more computationally efficient model. Along with the update gate, there exists another gate within the GRU, the reset gate, which helps to decide how much past information the model needs to forget.

GRUs have been quite effective in medical image analysis tasks involving sequential data. For example, a series of medical images could be used to track the progression of some diseases. Their features also lend themselves to scenarios that are computationally efficient, speedy, and therefore applicable—for example, real-time monitoring of patient vitals or continuous data streams from wearable medical devices. Such methods, like GRUs, can be applied not only to medical image captioning, which generate concise and relevant descriptions by processing sequences of image features.

6.3.3 Bidirectional RNNs

Bidirectional RNNs [27], belong to the category of recurrent neural network processing sequences in both forward and backward directions; therefore, there exist two hidden states for every time step. These capture information from the past and future context, hence developing a richer understanding of the sequence.

Bidirectional RNNs in medical imaging are useful for tasks that require context from the ends of the sequence. On this note, a bidirectional RNN will have better information about a complete cardiac cycle, considering the beginnings and the end of echocardiogram sequences in analyzing them. This approach, therefore, improves the accuracy of anomaly detection and assessment of heart function. This bidirectional RNN can make the results for the generation of medical reports further outstanding, giving a more holistic view of the image sequence and hence more accurate and full details of the reports.

6.3.4 Sequence-to-Sequence Models

Seq2Seq models [28], are a class of neural network architectures specially designed for tasks in which the input and output are sequences. Normally, a pair of encoders and decoders form them; this might be either RNNs, LSTMs, or even GRUs. Whereas an encoder is used to convert an input sequence into a context vector, the decoder is used to generate an output sequence from that vector.

Taking medical imaging to an even higher level are the structured and detailed reports given by Seq2Seq models. An example is that the encoder can process a sequence of medical observations, or features can be previously extracted from an image, such as a sequence of slices of a 3D MRI or even an ultrasound time-series data. At this level, the decoder will be able to generate a medical report to correspond with the given image. Complicated image data will be changed to a text file that is easily readable. The automation will put fewer workloads to the radiologists and make the report turnaround time better. It will summarize the most important findings and suggest possible diagnosis and require further tests with the help of the Seq2Seq model to help clinicians for proper action to be taken.

6.3.5 Transformer Models

Transformer models [29], are architectures that manage dependencies across long-range sequences lacking any recurrent structure. They adopt an encoder-decoder approach, and each of the elements involves self-attention and feed-forward layers. The self-attention mechanism determines the relative importance among different elements of the input to make the weight dynamically.

Transformers, by instance, have emerged as models that are capable of learning complex data dependencies and, thus, are revolutionizing medical report generation. In transformers, all sequences are processed at one go rather than sequentially, hence much faster and more efficient in processing. Because of the self-attention mechanism, transformers can capture relationships between different parts of the input sequence. This helps in improved context understanding—a major requisite in generating medical reports. Transformers provide a more coherent and contextually accurate report by dynamically centering more on the important sections of the input data. For instance, a transformer model in radiology can generate detailed descriptions of abnormalities found in various regions of an X-ray or CT scan. Multimodal Integration: Transformers can process multivariant inputs very easily and fuse them together to generate single output, i.e., it can integrate, say, image data with the patient's history or the lab results into the report being generated.

6.4 Applications of RNN and CNN in Medical Imaging

6.4.1 Sequence Analysis in Medical Imaging

Although the recording and analysis of temporal dynamics in most of the medical imaging modalities are essential. For instance, the heart's motion is observed over time during echocardiography, and temporal patterns of such motion are important for making diagnoses for heart abnormalities. Such temporal dynamics are well modelled using RNNs, through the hidden state and learning over the dependence over time steps. In sequences of image frames, RNNs can identify abnormalities produced in a motion pattern, such as irregular heartbeats or valve dysfunctions.

MR and CT volumetric data typically consist of many slices, which need to be analyzed contextually. RNNs can process sequences of slices while working out both spatial and temporal dependencies that are important for the accurate detection and segmentation of anatomical structures and pathological regions. For example, adjacent slices' arrangement relationships are taken into consideration by RNNs when determining and segmenting tumors in brain imaging.

6.4.2 *Image Captioning and Report Generation*

- Automatic Generation of Medical Reports
- This emerges to be one of the promising applications of RNNs in medical imaging. Radiologists and clinicians must put a lot of effort into analyzing medical images, making reports, and sometimes making lengthy detailed reports. RNNs, especially combined with CNNs, can automate this procedure. CNNs are used to extract features from medical images, and RNNs, more specifically LSTMs or GRUs, establish a coherent and contextually accurate textual description. This would involve training the RNN to understand the relationships between image features and related medical terminology for which it then creates full-fledged reports describing the findings and diagnosis recommendations.
- Image Captioning
- RNNs also find applications in image captioning, in which the description of a sentence is generated for every medical image and hence quite useful to summarize findings in words. For instance, an RNN could be trained to generate a caption for an X-ray image in the following terms: "normal lung fields" or "presence of pulmonary nodules." That will help optimize radiologists' workflow and improve locative efficiency during medical image interpretation.

6.4.3 *Predictive Modeling and Risk Assessment*

- Modeling the Progression of Disease
- RNNs are exquisitely good at modeling disease progression with respect to time. In sequences of medical images taken at different times, RNNs can capture dynamics related to disease progression. For example, sequences of MRI images in oncology can let them learn the growth and spreading of tumors to understand the process of planning treatment and estimating prognosis. Similarly, in chronic disease management, RNNs can also be applied to changes in organ structure, or changes in function over time, by evidencing how the diseases progress, and it helps to make good judgments by the clinicians.
- Risk Assessment
- The implementation of RNNs provides opportunities for predictive modeling and risk assessment through the analysis of time-series data acquired from medical imaging. For example, an application for cardiology could process sequences of echocardiographic images with RNNs to predict the risk of adverse cardiac events. Ability to capture the overall temporal trend of heart motion, the RNN could detect incipient signs of conditions like heart failure or arrhythmias, hence actually leading to early interventions for better patient outcomes.

- Multimodal Data Integration
- RNNs are also more powerfully multimodal, with the integration of information from sources of different information, enhancing the accuracy and robustness in medical image analysis. Imaging data and EHR information have different information to describe a patient's condition. The RNNs process sequences of imaging data mixed with textual data from EHRs; with this, the model considers visual and clinical information while generating a prediction or report. This multimodal approach enhances the diagnostic accuracy and gives an all-around patient health description.
- Improvement in Image Segmentation and Classification
- The embedding of temporal and contextual information through RNN can also enhance certain operations, such as segmentation and classification of images. Traditional approaches to image segmentation often work on an image-to-image or slice-to-slice basis and are not sensitive to useful contextual information. Clearly, the segmentation process can be improved in terms of accuracy and reliability, processing with the RNN model sequence composed of the images, which in turn provides an understanding of the temporal context. For instance, RNN would enable a model to consider image or feature order, especially in classification tasks, which implies better discriminative power of the model between, let's say, benign and malignant classes.

6.5 Transfer Learning in Medical Imaging

Transfer learning [30] is a machine learning technique that applies to the tuning of a pre-trained model on some large dataset, which in turn helps improve performance in a domain-specific dataset. A model borrowed from knowledge obtained during initial training, this approach leads to improved performance on target tasks with fewer labeled examples while reducing training time. Transfer learning is a very important constituent of medical imaging as it bridges the gap between having limited annotated data and needing highly accurate models for various applications [31].

6.5.1 Pre-training on Large Datasets

Pre-training on datasets, such as ImageNet, leads to learning generic features such as edges, textures, and shapes to be learned. As the medical image consists of such features, these models work fine for medical tasks after fine-tuning. Since the model starts with pre-learned initial layers, training on the medical dataset happens faster, being much lighter on computational power for that matter.

6.5.2 Fine-tune for Specific Tasks

It is by fine-tuning that the pre-trained model finally adjusts to the specific characteristics of the medical image, e.g., contrast, or noise variation in MRI or CT scans. Fine-tuning may enhance the capability of a model that recognizes some patterns of importance for diagnosis in medicine—tumors, lesions.

6.5.3 Applications in Medical Imaging

Through transfer learning, detection of diseases, comprising cancer, is enhanced by the ability to further improve the model performance in identifying deviation from normal patterns in radiological images. This can be done on anatomical structures together with pathologic regions of images for either therapy or monitoring purposes. Furthermore, transfer learning allows for the classification of different tissue types and organs together with the states of diseases; hence, improved diagnosis systems.

6.6 Deep Reinforcement Learning in Medical Imaging

Deep reinforcement learning [32] combines deep learning with the principles of reinforcement learning, whereby an agent learns from an environment to maximize cumulative rewards through interaction. DRL works with problems meant for sequential decision-making and high-dimensional data environments. Deep reinforcement learning has revolutionized how processes are optimized, decisions are taken, and images are interpreted better in medical imaging.

6.6.1 Automated Image Interpretation

It learns to enable the detection of anomalies in medical images through feedback from the accuracy of the predictions made by the DRL models. They keep improving their performance through this feedback loop. In image-developing, DRL can optimize image quality by learning the best methods for noise reduction, increase of contrast, and artifact removal for clearer images to be diagnosed.

6.6.2 Segmentation and Annotation

The progressive decision making of the DRL models can be used interactively for the segmentation of medical images wherein, it decides which pixel corresponds to a certain structure. This feature is highly expected to be useful in a very complex and variable anatomical structure. DRL can guide radiologist in the annotation of the images, thus suggesting the region of interest or naming the structure and makes the annotation process faster and lessens the human error.

6.6.3 Planning and Monitoring of Treatment

In radiation therapy planning, DRL may help optimize the dose distribution because it learns from prior data, further customized to the special needs of any individual, in order to deliver an effective and safe treatment. Models in DRL can help in the planning and guidance of surgeries by learning an optimum path discovery and not hitting critical structures to help in enhancing surgical result.

6.6.4 Image Registration

DRL would learn the ideal transformation parameters to enhance alignment from images coming from different modalities, like MRI and CT. This will help integrate complementary information to get a complete view of the patient's condition. DRL would hence be applied in the alignment of images that have been acquired during different time points. This would be greatly useful towards progress monitoring related to the disease during treatment.

6.6.5 Real-time Analysis

DRL will facilitate dynamic imaging types like ultrasound or functional MRI since measures are continuously trained to adapt to new incoming data. Consequently, it will allow the possibility of changing clinical decisions and treatment plans on the fly. The DRL can bring further optimization to imaging protocols on the fly by analyzing the images being acquired for the best quality of images and the best possible diagnosis while minimizing the dose of radiation to the patient.

6.7 Role of Data Science in Digital Imaging

In the realm of digital imaging, enhancing and restoring image quality is paramount. Data science has revolutionized this field with sophisticated algorithms that address noise reduction, image super-resolution, and color correction. Taxonomy of the image processing algorithms is presented in Fig. 6.3.

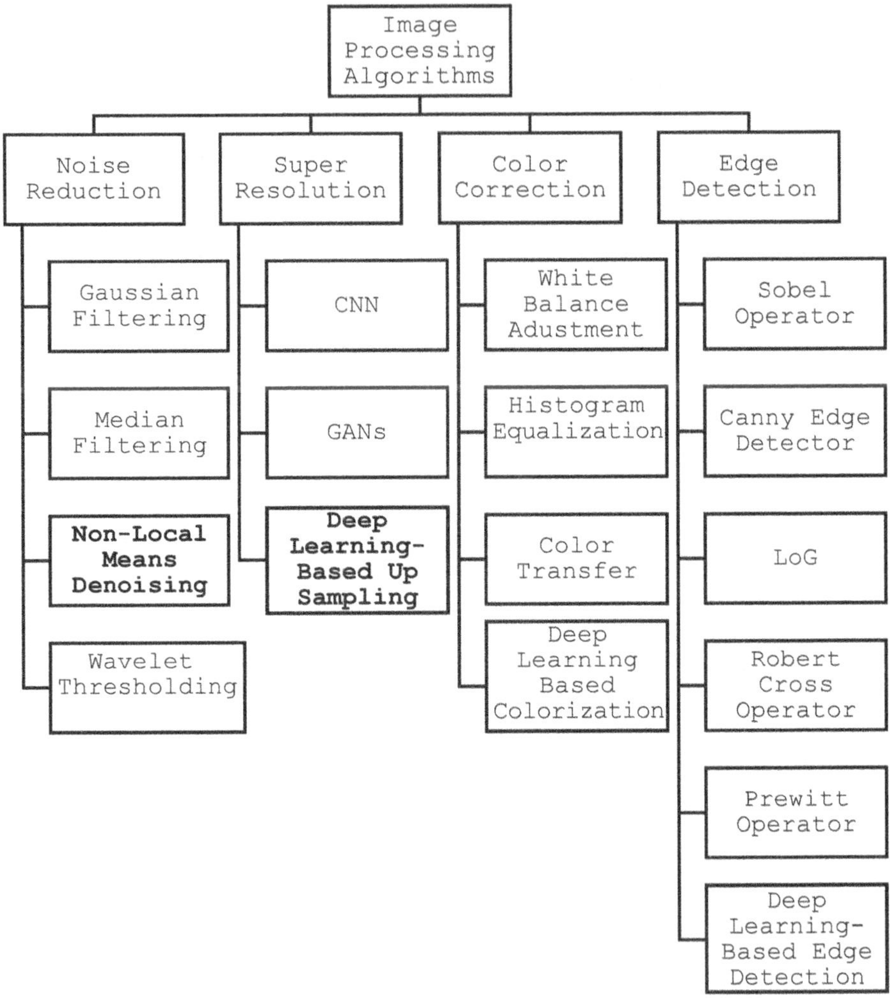

Fig. 6.3 Taxonomy of image processing algorithms used in data science

6.8 Image Processing Algorithms

6.8.1 Noise Reduction

Noise in digital images can originate from several sources, such as imperfections in the sensor of capturing device, environmental conditions, or transmission errors. Noise reduction is very important to have a clear and accurate image. So far, many algorithms have been developed for noise reduction, all with different strategies.

- Gaussian Filtering

- One of the essential techniques in noise reduction of images is Gaussian filtering [33]. The algorithm performs a Gaussian filtering that convolves an image with a Gaussian kernel, thus giving a smoothing effect by averaging pixel values with those of their neighbouring pixels. The Gaussian filter blurs the image, which reduces high-frequency noise but retains some details. This technique works quite well on Gaussian noise, but at the same time, it smoothens out edges and fine details.
- Median Filtering
- Median filtering [34] is a non-linear approach to filter salt-and-pepper noise, in which white and black pixels occur randomly. The algorithm replaces each pixel value with the median of pixel values in its neighbourhood.
- This method does not blur edges, since it selects a median value. It has many applications in image processing, more precisely in real-time noise reduction. Noise sometimes happens to be sporadic and extreme.
- Non-Local Means Denoising
- Non-local means denoising [35] is a sophisticated algorithm that works on the principle of comparing and averaging similar patches in the whole image, contrary to local filters. It includes information about patch similarity at different locations. Noises are efficiently removed while preserving textures and fine details by averaging patches with similar patterns. This technique has wide applications where high fidelity and texture preservation are required, including applications in high-resolution imaging.
- Wavelet Thresholding

- Wavelet thresholding [36] refers to the decomposition of an image into wavelet coefficients, thresholding these coefficients in a manner that reduces noise, and then reconstructing the image. The technique decomposes the image into different frequency components, thereby targeting noise reduction in this domain. Since the technique operates in the wavelet domain, it is very good at reducing noise while retaining features and edges. It works well with images that contain different levels of noise and fine details.

6.8.2 Super Resolution

The term super-resolution describes an increase in quality of an image above the quality of the individual images that make up this output. This is normally done for obtaining sharper and more detailed images from lower-resolution sources [37, 38].

- Convolutional Neural Networks (CNNs)
- Convolutional Neural Networks are the backbone of many state-of-the-art super-resolution approaches in use today. Models like Super-Resolution CNN (SRCNN) are trained with pairs of low-resolution and high-resolution images to learn the mapping from low to high resolution. Spatial patterns and features are learned during the training; hence, a high-resolution image from a low-resolution input can be generated using the same CNNs. This technique has very broad applications in digital imaging and computer vision, from the quality enhancement of images in consumer electronics to satellite imagery.
- Generative Adversarial Networks (GANs)
- Generative Adversarial Networks are applied in several techniques, such as SRGAN or Super-Resolution GAN, for generating high-resolution images. Here, GAN consists of a generator network that must be trained to generate a high-resolution image and another discriminator network that judges the quality of the generated images. Iterative improvements by the generator in generating more real images with details are due to the feedback received from the discriminator during the adversarial training process. GAN finds its applications in the creative field and practical applications that require high realism with fine details, such as art restorations and virtual reality.
- Deep Learning-Based Up Sampling
- Deep learning-based up sampling methods, especially EDSR, concentrate on the high-frequency details and residual learning. These networks perform image up sampling by refining the details of the image through residual connections to ensure the overall quality and resolution. Applications include mainly in cases where high quality images are derived from sources of low resolution, such as medical imaging and high-definition video.

6.8.3 Color Correction

Color correction ensures that the colors in an image are accurate, besides being aesthetically consistent. Sophisticated algorithms have been developed for adjusting colors to correct the distortions and achieve desired color effects.

- White Balance Adjustment
- White balance adjustment [39] algorithms correct color casts introduced by different lighting conditions so that white objects remain neutral. Various tech-

niques, ranging from simple assumptions of the gray world to more sophisticated techniques, are used. Colors are adjusted by the algorithm according to the estimated color temperature of the light source and hence show a natural appearance in an image. This method is used in the photography and video production industries to create a natural color appearance under various lighting conditions.

- Histogram Equalization
- Histogram equalization [40] is a method that modifies image contrast by readjusting the intensity levels of the image. The details in the bright and dark parts of an image become more vivid. This principle spreads the intensity values over the whole range, resulting in improved contrast and brightness. This has no flaws when it comes to the correction of under/overexposed images; therefore, it's very useful in medical imaging and scientific research.
- Color Transfer
- The algorithms of color transfer modify an image's color distribution to exactly match a reference image. Some common ways through which this is done include histogram matching and some other learning-based methods. Transfers the color characteristics of the reference image to the target image, balancing color imbalances or attaining certain color tones. Application: It could be of use in artistic applications, color grading for film, and enhancing visual consistency across images.
- Deep Learning-Based Colorization
- Colorization algorithms using deep learning, such as those in DeOldify, would colorize grayscale images or correct color imbalances. Such models learn from large datasets in a self-supervised manner to apply realistic colors to monochrome images. Trained neural networks on colored images to predict and apply colors to grayscale images for a plausible result. This approach gets applied in restoring historical photos and enhancing black-and-white films. The algorithms, in medical imaging, are supposed to enhance the resolution of the images acquired from MRI, CT, and ultrasound machines, thereby reducing diagnostic errors due to noise interference.

6.8.4 Edge Detection

Edge detection is a basic technique in image processing, which helps identify the boundaries and some of the important features of an image. A lot of algorithms are in use to detect edges, each with its own peculiar approach and application.

- Sobel Operator
- The Sobel operator [41] is another traditional way of edge detection; the operator computes the gradient of image intensity at each pixel. It uses convolution with Sobel kernels to detect edges in the horizontal and vertical directions. Computes

gradient magnitude and direction to highlight areas of rapid intensity change. Has broad applications in image processing, object detection, and feature extraction.
- Canny Edge Detector
- The Canny edge detector [42] is a multistep algorithm: first, Gaussian smoothing; then, gradient calculation; after that, non-maximum suppression; and lastly, edge tracking by hysteresis. The Canny detector was designed for the detection of a wide range of edges in images with high accuracy. It makes use of gradient magnitude and direction to detect edges, and hysteresis in tracing them accurately. Applications: Known for its precision, it is frequently used in computer vision tasks such as image segmentation and object recognition.
- Laplacian of Gaussian (LoG)
- The LoG [43] approach combines a Laplacian operator with smoothing, done by a Gaussian filter. A Gaussian filter smoothes the image first, and afterward this preprocessed image is applied to compute the Laplacian to find regions with rapid changes in intensity. It uses second-order derivative information towards edge detection with least noise. It is good for edge detection in noisy images and where accurate edge location is required.
- Roberts Cross Operator
- The Roberts Cross operator [44] detects edges by finding the differences in pixel values in the diagonal directions. The operator uses Roberts kernels, Similar to that of the Sobel operator, it emphasizes the diagonal edges by calculating gradient components in the x and y directions. This operator is particularly useful in applications where edge detection needs a simple and efficient method for highlighting the diagonal edges.
- Prewitt Operator
- The Prewitt operator [45] represents a modification of the Sobel operator, only using other convolution kernels for edge detection. It calculates gradients in the horizontal and vertical directions for finding edges. Compute gradient magnitude for edge detection, but with kernels specially designed to have high responses to edges in certain directions. In many image processing applications, like edge detection and feature extraction.
- Deep Learning-Based Edge Detection

- Deep learning edge detection techniques learn and detect edges using convolutional neural networks (CNNs) from the training data. Such methods use large datasets to improve the accuracy of edge detection and adapt to different image types. A technique that trains neural networks on ground truth images to learn complex patterns of edges and detect edges efficiently with high accuracy. Applied in state-of-the-art applications of Computer Vision, Scene Understanding, and Object Recognition.

6.9 Computer-Aided Diagnosis Systems

6.9.1 Detection Algorithms

These algorithms allow CAD to randomly locate abnormalities or markers of disease within medical images. Deep learning architectures and configurations, particularly convolutional neural networks, are among the most popular and widespread techniques used in the field of pathology for pattern recognition. For instance, CAD systems help identify entities related to breast cancer on mammograms, increasing the rate of diagnosis accuracy and patient recovery.

6.9.2 Classification Algorithms

These algorithms basically categorize medical images into different classes based on the extracted features or patterns. SVM, random forests, and neural networks are widely applied in this domain. In use, these algorithms not only classify an image into benign or malignant categories but also help in disease staging and determine the priorities of patient care by identifying critical cases that require immediate attention.

6.9.3 Decision Support Systems

Decision support systems incorporate the results of detection and classification algorithms to create actionable results for healthcare providers. One such system uses imaging data in conjunction with clinical information to provide diagnostic recommendations, suggestions of treatment options, and prognosis predictions. Such capability helps individualize medicine, optimizes workflow efficiency, and can refine strategies for the management of patients in radiology and beyond.

6.10 Data Mining Techniques

6.10.1 Association Rule Mining

Association rule mining realizes the relationships and dependencies among variables within these large medical image datasets. Apriori [46] and FP-Growth algorithms extract frequent patterns that allow determination of the associations co-occurrences of radiological findings or correlations between imaging biomarkers that help in understanding mechanisms of diseases, guiding further research, and refining diagnostic protocols.

6.10.2 Clustering Algorithms

This is a batch of algorithms that groups medical images with similar features, such as intensities, textures, or shape characteristics. Algorithms like k-means and hierarchical clustering enable unsupervised analysis, uncovering hidden patterns and subgroups in patient cohorts. Clustering helps in personalization of treatment plans for patients, stratification in clinical trials, and health interventions in populations.

6.10.3 Anomaly Detection Algorithms

These are methods for anomaly detection that outline the outliers or deviation from normal patterns, which may indicate some abnormality or rare conditions. Isolation forests, one-class SVMs, and deep autoencoders are some of the techniques applied in detecting subtle anomalies which might have usually been missed by other traditional methods. This capability aids in early disease detection, surveillance of disease progression, and monitoring treatment responses.

6.10.4 Predictive Modeling

Models of Regression Analysis for Predicting Continuous Clinical Variables: The relationship between imaging features and continuous clinical variables. For example, tumor size, patient's age, or physiological parameters can be predicted by models of regression analysis. Linear, polynomial, and ridge regression predict the outcome and the effect of imaging biomarkers on the progression of the disease. Predictive models inform treatment decisions, prognostic assessments, and therapeutic response assessments in clinical practice.

Classification models for predicting binary/categorical outcomes: These models identify binary or categorical outputs representing either the presence or absence of a disease or the staging of the disease based on imaging features and other data derived from the patient. Here, logistic regression, decision trees, and ensemble methods like gradient boosting classifiers help in the stratification of risk with accuracy for the management of patients. Such models allow interventions early in the process, treatment planning at the bedside of the patient, and prediction of outcomes in oncology, cardiology, and neurology.

Survival analysis methods evaluate imaging biomarkers with respect to their effects on patient survival as a function of time. Specifically, censored data is analyzed using Cox proportional hazards models, Kaplan-Meier estimators, and accelerated failure time models while accounting for different durations of follow-up. Such techniques allow for the prediction of the rate of recurrence of the disease, progression-free survival, and overall survival rates. These can help therapeutic strategies, patient counsel, and improvement of clinical trial design.

6.10.5 Natural Language Processing (NLP)

- Text Mining Algorithms
- Algorithms used in text mining are then applied to obtain structured information, like radiology findings or clinical notes, from unstructured medical reports. Among these natural language processing techniques, in particular, tokenization, NER, and sentiment analysis consider the challenges in rendering textual data into meaningful and actionable insights. NLP increases information retrieval, helps clinical decision-making, and enables secondary use of healthcare data for further activities in research and quality improvement initiatives.
- Named Entity Recognition
- This requires identifying and classifying entities within the medical text about anatomical terms, medical conditions, and treatment modalities. Advanced NLP models, especially bidirectional transformers such as BERT and clinical BERT, bring state-of-the-art performance in the recognition of domain-specific entities. This capability accelerates information extraction from EHRs, offers support in clinical coding, and enables interoperability between healthcare systems.
- Sentiment Analysis Techniques
- Sentiment analysis techniques assess emotion and subjectivity within narratives of patients, physicians' notes, and healthcare reviews. The machine learning models used are deep neural networks and support vector machines that perform the quantification of sentiment polarity, including positive, negative, and neutral, and their intensity levels. Products of sentiment analysis will inform patient satisfaction surveys, health-care provider feedback, and sentient-aware applications for improving patient-centered care.

6.11 Future Directions of Digital Imaging

Digitized imaging is an ultra-fast-moving area of development, as it gets pushed and pulled by equally rapid improvements in technology and novel applications across industries. The present chapter talks about new emerging technologies, future predictions, and their possible impacts on the user industries of digital imaging.

6.11.1 Artificial Intelligence and Machine Learning

Artificial intelligence and machine learning enable digital futures of imaging: increasing diagnostic accuracy, optimizing workflow efficiency for radiologists, and tailoring medicine. AI algorithms, brominated under the auspices of DL models and Neural Networks, have been intensely analyzing complex images of health and disease with accelerated speed and accuracy. Such technologies automate tasks related to image analysis and interpretation but find other hidden patterns and biomarkers that are useful in the very early detection of diseases and treatment planning.

6.11.2 D and 4-D Imaging

The transition from the conventional 2D imaging to 3D and 4D imaging modalities allows better spatial and temporal information to be conveyed to the clinician. Techniques of volumetric rendering, multi-planar reconstruction, and dynamic imaging document minute anatomical structures and physiologic processes in vivo. This will be much more helpful in many sub-specialties, especially cardiology, oncology, and orthopedics, where correct visualization along with navigation is key to both surgical planning and intervention.

6.11.3 AR and VR: Augmented and Virtual Reality

These technologies merge physical and digital worlds to allow for, amongst others, immersive medical training, surgical navigation, and patient education. AR overlays will supersede 3D visualization in the representation of patient-specific anatomy to improve accuracy and lower operative time during procedures. VR simulations develop skills and proficiency for complex procedures on the part of trainees in a risk-free environment.

6.12 Predictions for the Future

6.12.1 Artificial Intelligence in Clinical Workflows

This will become a standard integration of AI-driven tools and decision support systems within the clinical workflow. Continuously, AI algorithms will analyze vast imaging data, patient records, and genomic information to present real-time insights on personalized treatment strategies. Predictive analytics and machine learning models will predict progression, responses, and patient outcomes, ultimately changing the fabric of clinical decision-making forever and ensuring quality in patient care.

6.12.2 Advancements in Precision Medicine

Digital imaging will lead the way toward accelerating precision medicine efforts. Coupling the resolution of imaging modalities to genomic data allows tailoring of therapies based on genetics and features of disease processes. Radio genomics, by coupling detailed relations between imaging phenotypes to genomic data, will open a new armamentarium of disease diagnosis and prognosis biomarkers that will allow for targeted therapies and tailored treatments. Quantum Imaging and Nanotechnology.

Quantum imaging and nanotechnology are emerging technologies that have the promise of new breakthroughs in sensitivity, resolution, and contrast enhancement. Quantum sensors and nanoprobes enable ultrahigh resolution imaging of cell and molecular processes in all aspects of in vitro and in vivo studies. Thus, the possibility is created for early diagnosis of diseases at a molecular level, which will have far-reaching implications for cancer diagnosis, drug delivery systems, and biomedical research applications.

6.13 Potential Impacts on Various Industries

6.13.1 Healthcare and Medical Imaging

Advanced digital imaging technologies is going to bring efficient workflows, reduced diagnostic errors, and better patient outcomes in healthcare. AI-driven diagnostics and telemedicine applications will make specialized care reachable in far-flung areas, hence expanding health delivery for better patient satisfaction. Hence, digital pathology, molecular imaging, and wearable devices bring together an integrated ecosystem in personalized healthcare management.

6.13.2 Pharmaceutical and Biotechnology

The pharmaceutical companies will digitally enable their imaging technologies to accelerate drug discovery, optimize clinical trials, and monitor treatment responses. AI algorithms would analyze imaging biomarkers for stratification of patient populations, identification of therapeutic targets, and real-time evaluation of drug efficacy. Virtual drug screening and pharmacokinetic modeling that 3D imaging data enables will expedite the development of novel therapies against complex diseases.

6.13.3 Automotive and Manufacturing

It will also lead to innovation outside healthcare in the field of automotive safety, manufacturing quality control, and augmented reality applications. Autonomous vehicles use advanced imaging sensors and computer-vision systems that help such vehicles navigate complex environments with precision and reliability. Advanced 3D imaging methods are applied in manufacturing to monitor product quality, increase the efficiency of production, and even offer maintenance remotely.

6.14 Challenges and Ethical Issues in Digital Imaging

6.14.1 Image Quality and Standardization

One of the large challenges of digital imaging is related to ensuring that image quality is consistent for a given modality and among various healthcare facilities. Equipment differences, preparation methodology, and technical skill will have an impact on accuracy and reliability in the diagnosis in question. Professional organizations indeed have guidelines about this and support quality assurance programs to dampen the aforementioned challenges and optimize reproducibility in imaging.

6.14.2 Integration and Interoperability of Data

Integrating radiological images, pathology slides, molecular imaging data, and other such diversified sources of imaging creates interoperability challenges. The challenges stem from information silos, incompatible formats, and unstandardized metadata that lower further exchange and complete coordination of care. The interoperability frameworks and HIE seek to advance the integration of information to better coordinate patient care and collaboration in research amongst disciplines.

6.14.3 Technological Complexity and Its Adoption

The rapid evolution of digital imaging technologies, from artificial intelligence algorithms and advanced imaging modalities to associated system complexities in implementation, training, and maintenance, leads to the predicament of healthcare providers' acquisition and deployment of state-of-the-art technologies. In conjunction with this, there are a number of regulatory issues and workforce readiness.

In this regard, continuous education and clinical validation studies through strategic partnerships become all the more relevant to surmount technological barriers to the fullest and maximize the benefits of innovation.

6.14.4 The Privacy and Security of Patient Data

The protection of patient information and data security has become very critical in the case of digital imaging. Sensitive medical information will be stored in electronic health records, imaging archives, and cloud storage solutions that are always prone to breaches or unauthorized access—some even to cyber-attacks. It is important to ensure that health data privacy regulations, such as HIPAA in the US and GDPR in Europe, are applicable; that effective encryption, access controls, and audit trails for legal compliance on health data privacy rest within these guidelines to protect the integrity of patient data and preserve trust in healthcare systems.

6.14.5 Informed Consent and Patient Autonomy

Procedures for informed consent in imaging describe to the patient real risks, benefits, and alternatives. Meaningful consent to be achieved may be challenged by complex medical terminology, time constraints, and comprehension levels of the patients. It creates an obligation on the part of healthcare providers to ensure transparent communication, respect for the autonomy of patients, and address cultural and linguistic barriers in the informed decision-making process. Sharing decision making and protection of rights at all levels of the imaging continuum is underpinned by ethical guidelines and patient advocacy efforts.

6.14.6 Algorithm Bias and Clinical Validity

AI algorithms for use in digital imaging—in particular, machine learning models used for diagnosis or treatment planning—may be biased either by differences or biases in training data or internal to the algorithm. This may result in greater inadvertent biases, falling more heavily on underserved populations, increasing healthcare delivery and subsequently health outcome inequities. Ensuring a lack of bias in algorithms involves having diversified and representative training data sets, rigorous algorithm validation processes, and continuous monitoring for bias in practices.

6.15 Strategies to Address Ethical Concerns

6.15.1 Education and Training

Sustained education and training of all healthcare professionals, technologists, and data scientists are necessary for improving ethical sensitivity, updating knowledge of the latest clinical practices, and enhancing competence in the field of digital imaging. Curricula should include ethical reflections, regulatory provisions, and best practices for data handling, communication with patients, and transparency of algorithms. Collaboration among experts in the field of medical ethics, specialists in imaging, and technology developers leads to ethical decision-making and responsible innovation in healthcare.

6.15.2 Policy Development and Regulation

Government agencies, Health Organizations, and industry players are all in the development and enforcement of policies, standards, and guidelines that govern digital imaging practices. Some regulatory frameworks would therefore be of cardinal importance to keep all imagings within agreed ethical principles, data privacy laws, and standards of quality. Transparent reporting of AI algorithms with adherence to clinically validated protocols in aCallCheck of clinical validation protocols by robust governance frameworks ensures patient safety, mitigates risks, and promotes ethical accountability of digital imaging research and its clinical applications.

6.15.3 Stakeholder Engagement and Advocacy

Engagement of the patient, caregiver, advocacy group, and community stakeholders offers an avenue for inclusive dialoguing on concerns, value development, and practice in ethics for digital imaging. This will help set up patient-centered activities, open forums, and participatory research partnerships that stakeholders can leverage to express their views and influence policy and ethical guidelines. Ethical advocacy campaigns sensitize on patients' rights and data privacy issues and the social implications that emanate from emerging technologies, hence entailing trust and accountability within healthcare delivery.

6.16 Conclusion

Driven by digital imaging, the reshaping of health practices arises from characteristics that are typical of health innovation: technology advances, data-driven insights, and ethical considerations. It is in this setting that the chapter has tried to point out some ways data science is impacting digital imaging. Digital imaging algorithms enhance image quality by reducing noise, detecting edges, and segmenting the images, all of which are features that facilitate the diagnosis of many diseases using different modalities. CAD systems aid health professionals in detecting diseases automatically and improve workflow through advanced detection and classification algorithms. Some data mining techniques applied to these vast imaging data sets extract useful patterns that help in understanding mechanisms of diseases and treatment responses. It applies predictive modeling with regression and survival analysis using imaging biomarkers to predict clinical outcome, facilitating evidence-based decisions, while NLP strengthens the extraction and analysis of clinical insights from unstructured medical reports to improve coordination and quality of care.

The huge potential that emerging technologies in artificial intelligence, 3D and 4D imaging, and augmented reality hold for innovations in diagnostic and therapeutic strategies and possible future breakthroughs with precision medicine and quantum imaging have to be considered. At the very same time, however, challenges and ethical considerations like image quality standards, interoperability issues, and artificial intelligence complexities are some of the major concerns to be taken into consideration. Such strategies in terms of standardization, education, and policy-making must be designed to reduce biases and ensure equity in access to health care. About data handling and patient privacy, informed consent is a very serious ethical consideration for the maintenance of people's trust in health care systems. It is through responsible innovation, transparency, and stakeholder engagement that we can really exploit all the potential that digital imaging technologies can offer toward the advancement of patient-centered care and scientific discovery, thereby setting the future for healthcare delivery generations ahead.

References

1. P. Suetens, *Fundamentals of Medical Imaging* (Katholieke Universiteit Leuven, Belgium, 2017). Accessed 25 July 2024. [Online]. Available: https://books.google.com.pk/books?hl=en&lr=&id=U11EDgAAQBAJ&oi=fnd&pg=PA9&dq=medical+imaging&ots=vf_VScOsTj&sig=DqTHF5ozkb19Fz6rVc3cLmyNJ8o
2. K. Shung, M. Smith, B. Tsui, *Principles of Medical Imaging* (Academic, London, 2012). Accessed 25 July 2024. [Online]. Available: https://books.google.com.pk/books?hl=en&lr=&id=fUH_HrIHh30C&oi=fnd&pg=PP1&dq=medical+imaging&ots=yJ7iKTbLh0&sig=ohEQvNWMKMX9nDMvxfTPDn6cfBQ

3. R. Barua, J. Mondal, *Study of the Current Trends of CAD (Computer-Aided Detection) in Modern Medical Imaging* (IGI Global, 2023). igi-global.com. Accessed 25 July 2024. [Online]. Available: https://www.igi-global.com/chapter/study-of-the-current-trends-of-cad-computer-aided-detection-in-modern-medical-imaging/313470
4. S. Hussain et al., Modern diagnostic imaging technique applications and risk factors in the medical field: A review. Biomed. Res. Int. **2022**, 5164970 (2022). Wiley Online Library). https://doi.org/10.1155/2022/5164970
5. K. Yongmin, S.C. Horii, *Handbook of Medical Imaging. Volume 3, Display and PACS* (SPIE Press, Bellingham, 2000), p. 512. Accessed 11 July 2024. [Online]. Available: https://books.google.com/books/about/Handbook_of_Medical_Imaging.html?id=YKVULpCZ_iEC
6. S. Kiranyaz, O. Avci, O. Abdeljaber, T. Ince, M. Gabbouj, D.J. Inman, 1D convolutional neural networks and applications: A survey. Mech. Syst. Signal Process. **151**, 107398 (2021). https://doi.org/10.1016/J.YMSSP.2020.107398
7. D. Lu, Q. Weng, Q. Weng, A survey of image classification methods and techniques for improving classification performance. Int. J. Remote Sens. **28**, 823–870 (2007). https://doi.org/10.1080/01431160600746456
8. A. Krizhevsky, I. Sutskever, G.E. Hinton, ImageNet classification with deep convolutional neural networks. Commun. ACM **60**(6), 84–90. dl.acm.org (2017). https://doi.org/10.1145/3065386
9. U. Muhammad, W. Wang, S. Ali, S.P. Chattha, C.D.G. Khan, Pre-trained VGGNet architecture for remote-sensing image scene classification, in *2018 24th International Conference on Pattern Recognition (ICPR)*, (2018. ieeexplore.ieee.org). https://doi.org/10.1109/ICPR.2018.8545591
10. C. Szegedy et al., Going deeper with convolutions, in *Proceedings of the IEEE Computer Society Conference on Computer Vision and Pattern Recognition*, vol. 07–12-June-2015, (2014), pp. 1–9. https://doi.org/10.1109/CVPR.2015.7298594
11. S. Wu, S. Zhong, Y. Liu, Deep residual learning for image steganalysis. Multimed. Tools Appl. **77**(9), 10437–10453 (2018). https://doi.org/10.1007/S11042-017-4440-4
12. G. Huang, Z. Liu, L. van der Maaten, K.Q. Weinberger, Densely connected convolutional networks, in *CVPR*, (2017). openaccess.thecvf.com. Accessed 27 July 2024. [Online]. Available: http://openaccess.thecvf.com/content_cvpr_2017/html/Huang_Densely_Connected_Convolutional_CVPR_2017_paper.html
13. M. Tan, Q.V. Le, Efficientnet: Rethinking model scaling for convolutional neural networks, in *Proceedings of the 36th International Conference on Machine Learning, ICML 2019*, (Long Beach, 2019). Accessed 27 July 2024. [Online]. Available: http://proceedings.mlr.press/v97/tan19a.html?ref=jina-ai-gmbh.ghost.io
14. S. Ghosh, N. Das, I. Das, U. Maulik, Understanding deep learning techniques for image segmentation. ACM Comput. Surv. **52**(4), 40 (2019). https://doi.org/10.1145/3329784
15. N. Siddique, S. Paheding, C.P. Elkin, V. Devabhaktuni, U-net and its variants for medical image segmentation: A review of theory and applications. IEEE Access **9**, 82031–82057 (2021). ieeexplore.ieee.org. Accessed 11 July 2024. [Online]. Available: https://ieeexplore.ieee.org/abstract/document/9446143/
16. V. Badrinarayanan, A. Handa, R. Cipolla, SegNet: A deep convolutional encoder-decoder architecture for robust semantic pixel-wise labelling. IEEE Trans. Pattern Anal. Mach. Intell. **39**(12), 2481–2495 (2015). Accessed 11 July 2024. [Online]. Available: http://arxiv.org/abs/1505.07293
17. J. Sherrah, *Fully Convolutional Networks for Dense Semantic Labelling of High-Resolution Aerial Imagery* (arXiv:1606.02585, 2016). Accessed 11 July 2024. [Online]. Available: http://arxiv.org/abs/1606.02585
18. P. Bharati, A. Pramanik, Deep learning techniques—R-CNN to mask R-CNN: A survey. Adv. Intell. Syst. Comput. **999**, 657–668 (2020). https://doi.org/10.1007/978-981-13-9042-5_56
19. L.-C. Chen, G. Papandreou, S. Member, I. Kokkinos, K. Murphy, A.L. Yuille, Deeplab: Semantic image segmentation with deep convolutional nets, atrous convolution, and fully connected crfs. IEEE Trans. Pattern Anal. Mach. Intell. **40**(4), 834–848 (2017). ieeexplore.

ieee.org. Accessed 11 July 2024. [Online]. Available: https://ieeexplore.ieee.org/abstract/document/7913730/
20. B. Xu, F. Yang, J. Yang, S. Wu, Y. Shan, PNet: Superpixel pyramid network for scene parsing, in *2018 Chinese Automation Congress (CAC)*, (2018). ieeexplore.ieee.org. Accessed 11 July 2024. [Online]. Available: https://ieeexplore.ieee.org/abstract/document/8623025/
21. Y. Chen, M.C. Goorden, F.J. Beekman, J. Du, Understanding of object detection based on CNN family and YOLO. J. Phys. Conf. Ser. **1004**, 12029 (2018. iopscience.iop.org). https://doi.org/10.1088/1742-6596/1004/1/012029
22. R. Girshick, Fast r-cnn, in *Proceedings of the IEEE International Conference on Computer Vision (ICCV)*, (2015). openaccess.thecvf.com. Accessed 27 July 2024. [Online]. Available: http://openaccess.thecvf.com/content_iccv_2015/html/Girshick_Fast_R-CNN_ICCV_2015_paper.html
23. T.-Y. Lin, P. Goyal, R. Girshick, K. He, P. Dollar, Focal loss for dense object detection, in *Proceedings of the IEEE International Conference on Computer Vision (ICCV)*, (2017), pp. 2980–2988. openaccess.thecvf.com. Accessed 27 July 2024. [Online]. Available: http://openaccess.thecvf.com/content_iccv_2017/html/Lin_Focal_Loss_for_ICCV_2017_paper.html
24. J.M. Czum, Dive into deep learning. J. Am. Coll. Radiol. **17**(5), 637–638 (2020). https://doi.org/10.1016/j.jacr.2020.02.005
25. S. Hochreiter, J. Schmidhuber, Long short-term memory. Neural Comput. **9**(8), 1735–1780 (1997). ieeexplore.ieee.org. Accessed 27 July 2024. [Online]. Available: https://ieeexplore.ieee.org/abstract/document/6795963/
26. J. Chung, C. Gulcehre, K. Cho, Y. Bengio, *Empirical Evaluation of Gated Recurrent Neural Networks on Sequence Modeling* (arXiv, 2014). Accessed 27 July 2024. [Online]. Available: http://arxiv.org/abs/1412.3555
27. M. Schuster, K.K. Paliwal, Bidirectional recurrent neural networks. IEEE Trans. Signal Process. **45**(11), 2673–2681 (1997). ieeexplore.ieee.org. Accessed 27 July 2024. [Online]. Available: https://ieeexplore.ieee.org/abstract/document/650093/
28. I. Sutskever, O. Vinyals, Q.V. Le, Sequence to sequence learning with neural networks. Adv. Neural Inf. Proces. Syst. **27** (2014). https://doi.org/10.48550/arXiv.1409.3215
29. A. Vaswani, Attention is all you need. Adv. Neural Inf. Proces. Syst. **2017-December**, 5999–6009 (et al., 2017). Accessed 27 July 2024. [Online]. Available: https://arxiv.org/abs/1706.03762v7
30. M. Raghu, C. Zhang, J. Kleinberg, S. Bengio, Transfusion: Understanding transfer learning for medical imaging, in *33rd Conference on Neural Information Processing Systems (NeurIPS 2019), Vancouver, Canada*, (2019). proceedings.neurips.cc. Accessed 27 July 2024. [Online]. Available: https://proceedings.neurips.cc/paper/8596-transfusion-understanding-transfer-learning-for-medical-imaging
31. H.E. Kim, A. Cosa-Linan, N. Santhanam, M. Jannesari, M.E. Maros, T. Ganslandt, Transfer learning for medical image classification: A literature review. BMC Med. Imaging **22**(1), 69 (2020. Springer). https://doi.org/10.1186/s12880-022-00793-7
32. S. Zhou, Q. Wang, Deep reinforcement learning in medical imaging, in *Deep Learning for Medical Image Analysis*, (Academic, 2024). Elsevier. Accessed 27 July 2024. [Online]. Available: https://www.sciencedirect.com/science/article/pii/B9780323851244000106
33. K. Ito, K. Xiong, Gaussian filters for nonlinear filtering problems. IEEE Trans. Autom. Control **45**(5), 910–927 (2000). ieeexplore.ieee.org. Accessed 27 July 27, 2024. [Online]. Available: https://ieeexplore.ieee.org/abstract/document/855552/
34. B.I. Justusson, Median filtering: Statistical properties, in *Two-Dimensional Digital Signal Processing II. Topics in Applied Physics*, vol. 43, (Springer, Berlin/Heidelberg, 1981). Accessed 27 July 2024. [Online]. Available: https://link.springer.com/content/pdf/10.1007/bfb0057597.pdf
35. A. Buades, B. Coll, J.-M. Morel, Non-local means denoising. Image Process. **1**, 2011–2020 (2011. ipol.im). https://doi.org/10.5201/ipol.2011.bcm_nlm

36. M. Jansen, *Noise Reduction by Wavelet Thresholding* (Springer, 2012) Accessed 27 July 2024. [Online]. Available: https://books.google.com.pk/books?hl=en&lr=&id=WKTSBwAAQBAJ&oi=fnd&pg=PR12&dq=Wavelet+Thresholding&ots=D_CkfRDYYh&sig=E3wukZdT78SAg42Y6oXgTN46CfI
37. J. Tian, K.-K. Ma, A survey on super-resolution imaging. Signal Image Video Process. **5**(3), 329–342 (2011. Springer). https://doi.org/10.1007/s11760-010-0204-6
38. S. Anwar, S. Khan, N. Barnes, A deep journey into super-resolution: A survey. ACM Comput. Surv. **53**(3), 1–34 (2020). https://doi.org/10.1145/3390462
39. H. Lam, O. Au, C.-W. Wong, Automatic white balancing using adjacent channels adjustment in RGB domain, in *2004 IEEE International Conference on Multimedia and Expo (ICME) (IEEE Cat. No.04TH8763)*, (2004). ieeexplore.ieee.org, Accessed 27 July 2024. [Online]. Available: https://ieeexplore.ieee.org/abstract/document/1394366/
40. K.G. Dhal, A. Das, S. Ray, J. Gálvez, S. Das, Histogram equalization variants as optimization problems: A review. Arch. Comput. Methods Eng. **28**(3), 1471–1496 (2021). https://doi.org/10.1007/S11831-020-09425-1
41. N. Kanopoulos, N. Vasanthavada, R.L. Baker, Design of an image edge detection filter using the Sobel operator. IEEE J. Solid State Circuits **23**(2), 358–367 (1988). ieeexplore.ieee.org. Accessed 27 July 2024. [Online]. Available: https://ieeexplore.ieee.org/abstract/document/996/
42. L. Ding, A. Goshtasby (2001) "On the Canny edge detector," Pattern Recogn. 34(3), 721-725. Elsevier. Accessed 27 July 2024. [Online]. Available: https://www.sciencedirect.com/science/article/pii/S0031320300000236
43. Steve R. Gunn. On the discrete representation of the Laplacian of Gaussian, Pattern Recognit. **32**(8), 1463–1472 (1999). Elsevier. Accessed 27 July 2024. [Online]. Available: https://www.sciencedirect.com/science/article/pii/S0031320398001630
44. S. Al-Amri, N. Kalyankar, S.D. Khamitkar, Image segmentation by using edge detection. Int. J. Comput. Sci. Eng. **02**(03), 804–807 (2010). Citeseer. Accessed 27 July 2024. [Online]. Available: https://citeseerx.ist.psu.edu/document?repid=rep1&type=pdf&doi=1f2ac2b9ef743be79a40bcef23bfa3a5bf750b36
45. W. Dong, Z. Shisheng, Color image recognition method based on the prewitt operator, in *2008 International Conference on Computer Science and Software Engineering*, (2008). ieeexplore.ieee.org. Accessed 27 July 2024. [Online]. Available: https://ieeexplore.ieee.org/abstract/document/4723223/
46. M. Hegland, The Apriori algorithm—A tutorial, in *Mathematics and Computation in Imaging Science and Information Processing*, (2007), pp. 209–262. https://doi.org/10.1142/9789812709066_0006

Chapter 7
Public Health Surveillance and Resource Optimization

7.1 Introduction

The computing and communication technologies, in addition to managing physical and mental health of individuals, also promise to reshape the public health. According to WHO, public health surveillance can be defined as "continuous and systematic collection, orderly consolidation and evaluation of pertinent data with prompt dissemination of results to those who need to know, particularly those who are in a position to take action" [1]. In the past, data collection was limited to conventional methods, such as through conducting public events at clinics or public spaces. Moreover, the data was also frequently gathered using survey forms, which was again slow, costly and cumbersome. The conventional approach yielded a restricted amount of data and made it impractical to reach millions of citizens within a country. As a result, it was not possible to collect realistic data about health trends or disease prevalence among the population. Similarly, it was also a challenge to communicate the population health risks to the authorities due to the lack of analytics and visualization tools.

Using IoT, DS and AI, it has become possible to collect massive amount of data from large populations which leads to a significantly better opportunity for the state to get an insight into the actual statistics. Today we have advanced forms of data sources such as smart phones, wearable and ambient devices, social media, search histories and EHRs; all of these and others can be regarded as health surveillance data and can be fed into advanced data analytics systems [2]. Through the use of technology, not only the current population health state can easily be communicated to the authorities, but advanced ML algorithms also offer an opportunity to predict the possible diseases and their impact.

The technologies of IoT, DS and AI are not only used for managing population health but they also focus on healthcare resources such as staff and equipment. Almost all over the world, there is a shortage of medical professionals and

S. Siddiqui et al., *Connected Health Insights for Sustainable Development*,
https://doi.org/10.1007/978-3-031-81433-4_7

equipment; there is always a need to manage the available resource efficiently. The technologies discussed in this book offer help in this domain by providing a means of monitoring the patients as well as healthcare facilities in the real-time. At one hand, continuous patient monitoring reduces the chances of hospitalization/re-hospitalization and on the other hand, the facilities are being increasingly automated. For example, automated appointment systems and RFID-embedded equipment reduces the need of healthcare workforce.

This chapter describes some of the major techniques of IoT-DS-AI nexus which help to achieve effective public health surveillance and resource optimization.

7.2 IoT Collects Population Data

IoT appears as a simple yet cost-effective technology for collecting population health data. Wearable health monitors, smart watches, wristbands, environmental sensors and connected hospital equipment provide enormous amount of population health data. As discussed in the previous chapters, once the data enters the IoT-DS-AI nexus, it offers unlimited opportunities for analyzing health trends, predict patient outcomes and diseases and monitoring the effectiveness of health interventions. Thus, public health authorities can get an early insight into the population health risks and can engage in more effective intervention planning.

Various IoT applications were developed during COVID-19 period, due to the specific requirements of social distancing and quarantine management. Some example use cases of using IoT for managing population health are discussed in this section.

7.2.1 IoT During COVID

Various IoT solutions and centralized dashboards were developed during COVID to monitor the spread of virus, direction of spread and even the severity for affected people belonging from different regions, ages, medical backgrounds etc. In this context, not only the wearable devices, but also connected hospital systems come into play for providing a comprehensive health insight. At the US, Kinsa developed FDA approved smart thermometers which are generally used for monitoring flu and flu-like illnesses. The device could synchronize with a mobile app, which subsequently sends data to the company's dashboard. To maintain the user privacy, before transmission to the company's server, the data is anonymized. Before COVID, Kinsa thermometers were already in use to predict the spread of flu. During 2020 and later, these thermometers were used to assess the direction of COVID spread in various counties of the US. Also, novel applications for the Kinsa users were reported, for example, a study was conducted to identify the impact of children presence at home on the spread of COVID within the family [3]; another study focused on identifying the epi-center of COVID using connected thermometers provided by Kinsa [4]. This trend shows that not only IoT plays a major role in communicating the present health state to the authorities, but innovative insights can also be developed, which would in turn be useful for planning customized intervention based on the need of each family.

Due to the high number of patients, particularly at the regions with lesser medical workforce or infrastructure, wearable devices offered significant assistance in managing the pandemic. The patients with high risks were continuously monitored at their homes before hospitalization or after discharge. Such strategies did not only improve the survival rate for patients but also considerably reduced the burden on hospitals as the staff as well as beds fell short at most of the world. The most common parameters monitored remotely during COVID were temperature and pulse oximetry, however, in certain cases, remote ECG was also performed for managing higher risks of respiratory failures. Although, conventional ECG is taken by using patches on the chest, the product facilitating predictive algorithm-based wristband based ECG has also been made commercially available.

Travelling within and beyond countries was very limited during COVID-19 period. However, for the necessary travel, the airports made it mandatory for the passengers to bring negative PCR results and be in isolation for the first 3 days of their arrival. To still be safe from spread of COVID due to travel, various airports across the globe deployed IoT technology. For example, upon arrival, passengers were given RFID and GPS embedded wristbands [5]; in case the users leave from their designated quarantine locations, the authorities would know via central dashboard interfaces and the appropriate action could be taken. Moreover, RFID tags were also used for automated baggage handling systems and e-passports to prevent staff from coming into contact with the luggage or travel documents.

Contact-Tracing was another major concept emerged during the surge of COVID, just like social distancing and quarantine monitoring. Various companies developed Bluetooth enabled wristband and similar solutions that kept the record of who had come nearby the person who later got infected by the virus. These wristbands mostly connected to the mobile apps, which transmitted the data to centralized databases; such contact tracing measures were taken both at organizational and state levels [6]. Similarly, the wristbands also participated in maintaining social distancing; an alert was generated if a person came near to someone else.

At organizational level, various novel developments were made to control the spread of COVID. Innovative mobile apps were generated to remind about washing hands, keeping hands away from the mouth and maintaining social distancing. Alerts were also sent to the people if someone who had come near over the past week had developed COVID; this helped in detecting the suspicious cases so they could be advised to be at quarantine. IoT solutions also helped to trace the crowd while entering the premises of offices, markets or airports. Smart cameras and infrared sensors were used by the staff posted at the points of entry to detect the suspicious cases. Since high grade fever was the common symptom of COVID, the use of contactless infrared thermometers became the norm for quickly monitoring people.

7.2.2 *Mobile-Based Crowdsensing Platforms*

In Chap. 4 we discuss the paradigm of mobile health and the most commonly used mobile applications and digital platforms for various healthcare applications. However, mobile sensing can also serve as a population health management tool. Although the core underlying technologies such as wearable devices, cloud computing, mobility monitoring and mobile data offloading remains same for both domains of personalized and population health management, the goals are significantly different [7]. Various population health determinants about mental and physical health can be collected using mobile crowdsensing platforms, which can subsequently be used for developing predictive models. Some of the major areas in which mobile apps and sensing platforms can aid the population health surveillance include depression and anxiety monitoring, tracking sleep quality and insomnia patterns and assessing connection between human mobility and spread of epidemics Fig. 7.1 lists these applications and the discussion follows next.

- Pandemic/Epidemic Tracking
- The wearable devices as well as ambient sensors could provide a great insight into the degree to which population is at risk. As the use of IoT devices for COVID management has been discussed above, other pandemic and epidemics may also be tracked based on the vital parameters they affect. For example, Influenza can most easily be monitored as it causes fever and may affect respiratory rate and heart rate variability; all of these can be measured using cost-effective and easily available commercial devices. Ebola can be monitored as it also causes fever; the spread can be tracked and patients can be quickly isolated. Moreover, the ambient devices installed at the patient's home can also shed light on their health state, offering authorities with an opportunity to map the risks.
- The environmental sensors can also be used for detecting the risk of virus at the given regions. The presence of mosquitoes, temperature and humidity of the environment can help to predict the risk of Malaria, Dengue and other related

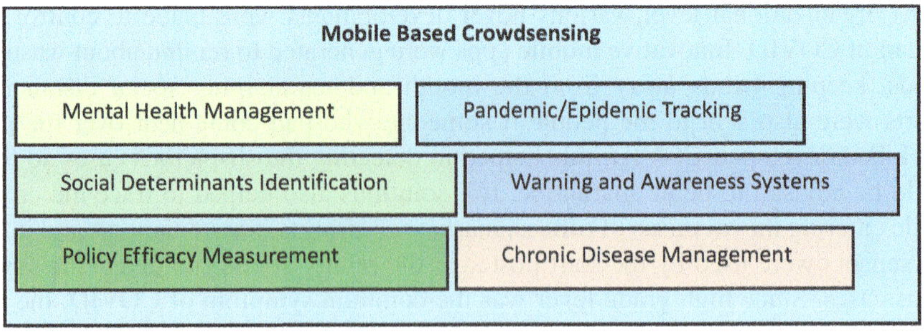

Fig. 7.1 Major applications of mobile-based crowdsensing for healthcare

viruses. Even Zika can also be predicted by detecting and studying the mosquito population dynamics.

- Mental Health Management
- Mobile based crowdsensing offers unique methods for assessing the mental health issues of population. Data from mobile apps, wearable devices (such as pulse rate sensors and SPO_2 monitors), ambient devices and social media usage is integrated together to identify the anxiety, depression and other mental health parameters, as earlier discussed in Chap. 4. Similar applications are also used for detecting the mental health issues of population and various approaches have been designed in this way. For example, data from user surveys designed based on standard psychological tools and wearable devices can be integrated to get a comprehensive insight into the mental health challenges; techniques of alternative medicines such as music therapy can be introduced based on the anxiety detection using wearable devices; sleep patterns of a population can be identified and its linkage with the occurrence of psychological issues can be studied.
- Various mobile apps targeting mental health issues, as already discussed in Chap. 4 provides community support. Elderly population all across the world are the most prone to developing anxiety, depression and other psychological disorders. Among many others, one of the major reasons is the lack of support system, as many of them are empty nesters and they develop sense of loneliness. Although there are community and religious centers often available for supporting them, but in the presence of situations such as epidemic or lack of access to such location because of residing at far-off areas, the mobile Apps, social media and IoT all come together for offering community support. Based on the social trait and risk assessment of elderly, relevant community support is offered through internet by suggesting other users who are similar in attributes. Thus, people can have a sense of human connectivity through using technology.
- Managing Chronic Diseases
- The massive data collected from participants using IoT wearable or ambient devices sheds light on the lifestyle patterns as well as medical and family history of the users. When such users are identified for suffering from chronic diseases such as hypertension, diabetes or cardiac issues, it becomes possible to find out the social determinants in a certain set of population. For example, it may be identified that population at a certain region is used to of sedentary lifestyles which might become the major reason behind obesity and cardiac diseases.
- The real-time monitoring and customized reporting which is the core functionality of IoT further adds value to the population health systems, when combined with alert generations. In case the values of vitals are found to be above threshold for the patients, alerts are generated for the patients, doctors and also other selected caregivers (such as family members). This functionality provides an opportunity to the physicians and care providers for identifying the users at risk and develop early intervention for them. For example, if many people belonging from a group with common social determinants are facing any chronic issues, the

medical experts and policy makers may approach others with the same attributes for early interventions. This would prevent a larger set of population from developing the same high risks for chronic diseases.

- Warning and Awareness Systems
- Generating timely alerts for informing the patients, caregivers and physicians has been one of the core reasons for using automated healthcare technologies. This includes the usual fitness monitoring and chronic disease management platforms for individuals as well as risk identification systems for the population. Many recent applications of alerts and warnings were seen during the COVID. At an individual level, the wristbands and mobile apps used to send alerts to the users in different situations: when their body temperature rose, when they were in the high-risk areas, when they were not maintaining the social distance, when they were not allowed to get outside due to quarantine etc. similarly, the central dashboards were used by organizations and state to study the patterns of COVID spread. For example, the hospitals used to enter the data about admission, death and re-occurrence of COVID patients, which was subsequently fed into the central dashboards for review of the decision-making authorities.
- In addition to generating warnings, the IoT based connected mobile apps also play a crucial role for generating population health awareness. In the past, these sessions were restricted due to physical access, schedule and cost. Today, the community health systems collect population data using IoT devices, do analytics and conduct online awareness sessions. For example, a population sector at a high risk of developing obesity and relevant diseases such as Diabetes type II may be scheduled for a session with diabetologists and fitness experts to raise awareness about the diet and exercise routines. The online awareness sessions increase access, reduce cost and at the same time, also develop the sense of community as the participants may motivate each other.
- Monitoring Policy Efficacy
- In addition to monitoring the health statistics of population, the mobile based sensing applications can also provide an insight into the effectiveness of the government's policies. For example, the technology was widely used during COVID-19, where the impact of government's policies regarding lockdown, social distancing, travel restriction and quarantine was monitored. Moreover, the degree of implementation of the policies was also measured using the same technology by monitoring the number of devices at home, and those at public places. Similarly, mobile app based survey can easily be conducted to identify the mental and physical health of population by taking their own feedback. The public satisfaction with the health-related policies of the government can quickly be identified using survey; this would not only improve the public trust on state, but would also offer the policy makers with a chance to integrate broader perspective in the future policies.

7.2.3 *Healthcare Resource Management*

The crucial resources of healthcare sector that include the workforce and healthcare inventory, equipment/facilities and medications can be optimized using real-time data obtained by IoT. Wireless sensors, tags and devices associated with medical equipment and facilities help to collect data and optimize usage and allocation of public resources. Eventually, the data is transmitted to the remote servers, from where policymakers can get access via comprehensive reports and graphs; this helps in allocating sufficient resources to each region. Some of the areas in which IoT plays an important role for resource management are highlighted in Fig. 7.2:

- Inventory Management
- Using connected sensors, hospitals can deploy smart shelves and cabinets for asset management. Such modern shelves automatically track the inventory levels of medical supplies, medications, and equipment, ensuring timely restocking and reducing waste. Moreover, RFID tags are often placed on assets and equipment to track their location. Smart refrigerators also contribute to the inventory management by maintaining and logging the required temperature by diverse medical supplies. All these initiatives help to collect real-time data about medical inventory, prevent loss and preventive maintenance.

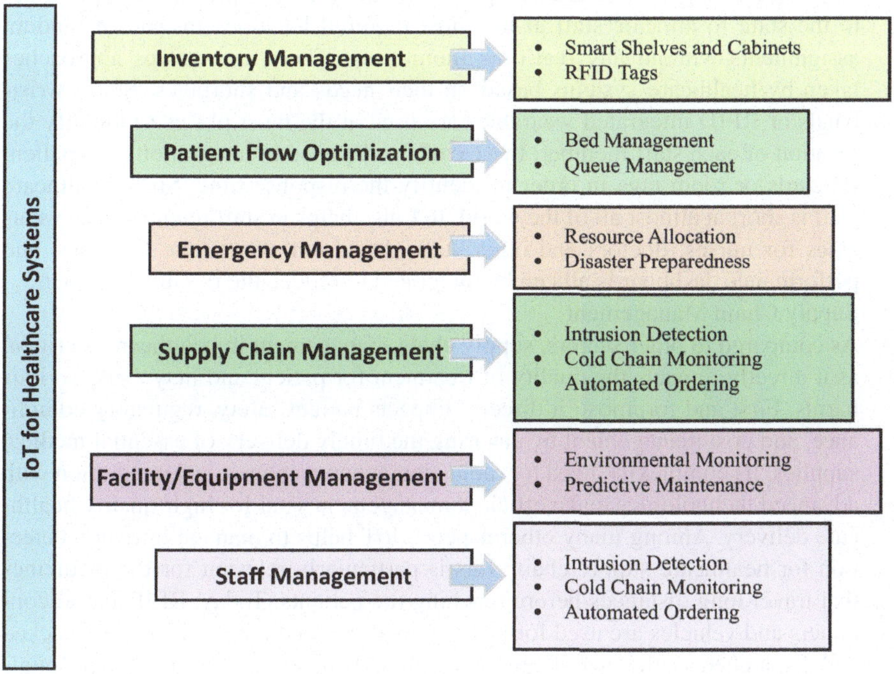

Fig. 7.2 Applications of IoT for public healthcare resource management

- Patient Management
- Bed management has been one of the first IoT application for the hospitals. Sensors are embedded with hospital beds which inform the centralized patient information systems as well as state authorities about the occupancy of each bed. The occupancy information helps to reduce the staff workload and improves the processes of discharge and admissions. Moreover, the sensors can also be deployed for informing about the malfunction of various components of bed, which reduces the downtime and improves the patient service quality.
- Also, patient flows are optimized using IoT devices as the patients are continuously monitored using wearables which reduces the need for hospital visits overall, and particularly the re-hospitalization rates [8]. Once the patients are at hospitals and they visit various departments such as Out Patient Department (OPD), diagnostic labs, X-rays, etc., their flow can be monitored using wristbands, RFID, cameras and location sensors. This also helps to identify the bottleneck process. As a result of these measures, hospitals need to manage shorter queues, result in cost-savings as the staffing needs are reduced. Automated check-ins have also been installed at various facilities, which reduces the queuing time as patients can check-in from multiple kiosks and even from their own mobile applications.
- Staff Management
- As discussed above, IoT facilitates inventory and patient flow management in a way that staffing need at each hospital is reduced, hence, providing opportunity to the state to allocate staff at the most required locations instead of random assignments without any real-time monitoring. There are various approaches taken by healthcare systems based on their needs and shortages. Smart wristbands or RFID integrated wearables are used at the most places to identify the location of each staff member; these can also be used in integration with patient ID cards or room tags in order to identify the response time. Since healthcare staff is short at almost all of the world, IoT also helps in staff retention; the wearables for nurses, doctors and other staff, data from smart time machines and performance dashboards all can be integrated to reduce the possible burnout.
- Supply Chain Management
- As compared to other sectors, supply chain management in healthcare is critical as it directly impacts the quality of treatment for patient and may cause serious harms. First and foremost, it directly impacts patient safety, regulatory compliance, and cost management by ensuring the timely delivery of essential medical supplies. Its complexity, need for rapid emergency response, and integration with advanced technologies make efficient management vital for high-quality healthcare delivery. Among many other aspects, IoT helps to manage intrusion detection for healthcare supply chain; this is particularly relevant for the medicines that travel long distances before reaching the patients. Today, RFID based containers and vehicles are used for ensuring that the medicines which were packed and dispatched by the manufacturers reach in their original form to the hospitals and patients. There is a high risk involved in case intrusion happens enroute and some medicine which do not satisfy the quality criteria or are expired are added

to the consignments. To avoid these, RFID technology is used and each package is checked by the readers at multiple locations to ensure that all the packages are intact and meet the quality standards. GPS sensors also help to identify the location of vehicles as well as to identify exact points where intrusion has taken place.

- Further to avoiding intrusions, it is also critical to ensure that medicines reach desired locations, while be in their required temperature range. Various medicines are categorized as per their requirement of having specific temperature ranges and the temperature should not go up or down the specified threshold else, they would not remain effective; for example, the medicines to be maintained at the temperature range of 2–8 °C should not be frozen. This process of maintaining the temperature of medicine products at the required values throughout the supply chain is referred as cold chain management. IoT temperature sensors collect real-time data about the temperature and send to the remote dashboards. The stakeholders may immediately know about the temperature variations and may arrange for alternative methods to protect the medicines. Moreover, there are also dataloggers present within the containers which keep all the record of temperature; these logs are then checked at the points of entry at distribution centers and pharmacies. In case the logs show that temperature had gone down or up during a journey, entire consignments worth thousands of dollars can be rejected, hence, guaranteeing patient safety.
- Automated ordering for medicines and medical supplies has also become possible due to the use of smart refrigerators, shelves and cabinets. When the sensors integrated with this equipment identify the shortage of supplies, they could place automatic orders. This reduces human intervention and streamlines the procurement process. At one hand, this technology ensures that the supplies never get short on shelves and remain available at the required time, on the other hand, it eliminates the problems of over-ordering and stocking of medicines and supplies. For example, this problem is often faced during the incidents such as COVID when people and private hospitals were stocking on necessary life saving medicine. In case IoT and relevant technologies are used, the state gets an insight about the exact point where problem is introduced in the system, leading to better administration.
- Facility/Equipment Management
- Using environmental sensors such as temperature and humidity, the healthcare facilities can be optimized to perform. For example, the lightning and cooling/heating systems can be monitored in real-time and can be remotely operated to reduce the energy consumption. Cameras and proximity sensors can also be used in integration with environmental sensors to further automate the facility management. Various logics can be designed in smart healthcare facility management scenario; if there is no one present at a facility, the cooling/heating system may be shut down despite the temperatures.
- IoT also serves well for healthcare equipment management, again due to the basic functionality of real-time monitoring. The use of vibration, pressure, flow, gas, load and position sensors have been common for industrial equipment moni-

toring. The sensors relevant to hospital equipment are now used to inform about the need of repair and identification of expected malfunction due to the routine wear and tear such as rusting. When informed timely, the hospital authorities may timely replace or repair the equipment which improves the service quality. If the need be, the hospitals can request state authorities for the procurement of new equipment well in advance, instead of waiting for actual crash to happen. At the level of state, this will not only reduce the cost of repair, but would also reduce the risks for patients. As ideally, all the hospitals should be connected, the state will also have information if similar equipment is lying underused or unused at some other location, it can also be relocated to the place where it is most needed.

- Emergency Management
- Disaster and emergency response planning is one of the core responsibilities of the state healthcare authorities. With the help of connected devices and systems feeding data into central dashboards, it becomes possible for the authorities to identify the best suited locations for offering care to those affected by the disaster/emergency. Just like the patients, the healthcare staff can also be allocated to the location with the most patient influx, rather than staying idle at their regular workplace. The ambulance drivers can also be tracked and sent alert about the locations they must reach; in this context, the handheld devices of drivers and GPS trackers of vehicles come into play. It becomes possible for the authorities to route the nearby ambulances to the affected location which improves the chances of survival of the affected by reducing the response time.
- The state can be better prepared for dealing with disasters with the help of IoT. As discussed above, the authorities are regularly updated about the factors such as bed occupancy, equipment malfunction and shortage of staff. Based on this data, the policymakers can easily assess their capacity to accommodate casualties in case some disaster happens. For example, if 80% of the healthcare resources remain occupied all the time under normal circumstances, the planning division might need to allocate more budgets to develop more healthcare infrastructure to deal with emergencies.

7.3 Data Science for Population Health Analytics

With the massive volumes of data available, population health management has become easier than never before. These systems have three major tasks: collecting and integrating data from multiple sources, applying best suited analytics to the collected data and providing the required care to the population through appropriate policy development and implementation.

7.3.1 Data Integration

As discussed in Sect. 1.7, the second level in the IoT-DS-AI nexus is DS, which takes data from the IoT devices. Although due to availability of electronic health, it has become easier and practical to gain quick insights into population health trends, there is a need of integrating data obtained from multiple sources. Previously, there was no concept of continuous data streams flowing through wearable/ambient sensors or mobile apps; all data available used to be the medical history of patients available with their doctors; however, now we have distributed system of health data generation, with significantly increased number of stakeholders. Data is generated by separate hospitals, clinics, diagnostic centers and patients' devices; all sources claim ownership of their data and often do not share even with the patients. This is particularly valid for the developing and under-developed countries where it is more critical to develop and implement laws governing data ownership and sharing. Therefore, there is a need to integrate health data generated from various points in order to develop a clear picture of the patient health both at individual and population level. The key steps used for data integration in the healthcare domain facilitated by DS are shown in Fig. 7.3:

Data Science has developed various tools for data integration simplifying the interpretation for healthcare stakeholders. Some of the examples of data integration tools include Talend, Informatica, Apache NiFi, and Microsoft Azure Data Factory. These tools provide built-in functionalities for data extraction, transformation, and loading, as well as for handling complex data integration workflows. While integrating data from various sources, it is also crucial to manage the synchronization. DS tools set up processes for regularly updating the integrated data and resolving any discrepancies that may arise between the source systems and the integrated repository.

7.3.2 Population Risk Identification

Through applying data science, the governments are mainly interest to develop their health contingency plans to deal with any emergencies. These plans aim to ensure that healthcare systems can continue to operate effectively during events such as

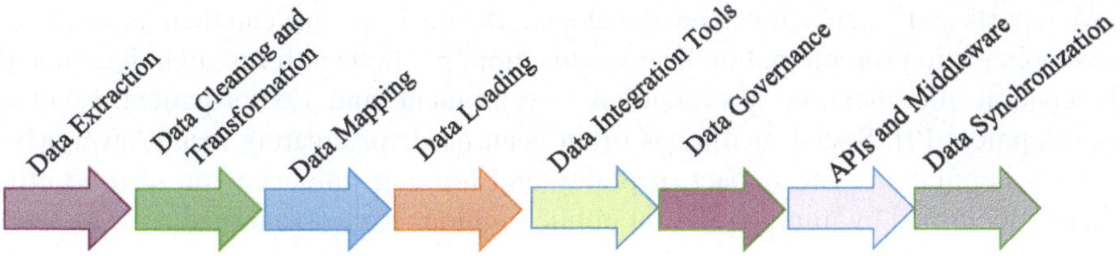

Fig. 7.3 Data integration for population health using data science

pandemics, natural disasters, bioterrorism attacks, or other public health emergencies. The key components of health contingency planning served by data science include predictive analytics through using ML models and simulations, resource allocation, and managing public health surveillance measures. DS also supports to identify the impact of emergency/disaster by providing large scale data.

As discussed above, collecting data from multiple population sectors help the authorities to define certain population groups. For example, some population groups can be defined based on their risks towards chronic diseases or viruses. Subsequently, the risks are stratified based on the risk level of each patient; this helps to further narrow down the risk assessment and prioritize the patients for their hospital visits, hospitalizations etc. Thus, risk assessment and population categorization takes place. Next, based on the risk stratification, the reports and visualization are produced for communication with all the stakeholders including policy makers. Finally based on the risk assessments, the governments allocate resources to each sector according to their demographic assessment of the population health risks.

7.3.3 *Social Media and Health Data Analytics*

Social media has emerged as a major source of big health data. Data analytics are increasingly being performed over social media data which help to identify public health trends, disease outbreaks, patient experiences, and perceptions about/satisfaction with healthcare delivery. As a first step, health-related information, opinions, and experiences are collected through various social media platforms like Twitter, Facebook, Instagram, and Reddit; APIs (e.g., Twitter API) and web scraping are often used for this extraction. Next step is data processing, as people use natural language to write their opinions on social media; therefore, to infer the relevant information, text preprocessing steps, including tokenization, stop-word removal, stemming, and lemmatization, are applied to clean the data. Moreover, multi-language content can be dealt with by using language detection and translation services. For data analysis, the techniques of Natural Language Processing, Statistical Analysis, Predictive Modeling and visualization are often used for social media health related analytics; these techniques are summarized in Fig. 7.4:

Data analytics performed over social media posts helps the authorities to gain knowledge about disease surveillance and public perceptions. Once the comprehensive reports and visualizations are developed, the governments can then make effective policies to promote public health education, public health research, health and behavioral modification, professional development and doctor-patient relation development [9]. Social media has often been used for creating health awareness among population. The impact of policy and training influence can also be efficiently identified by mining relevant public opinions from social media.

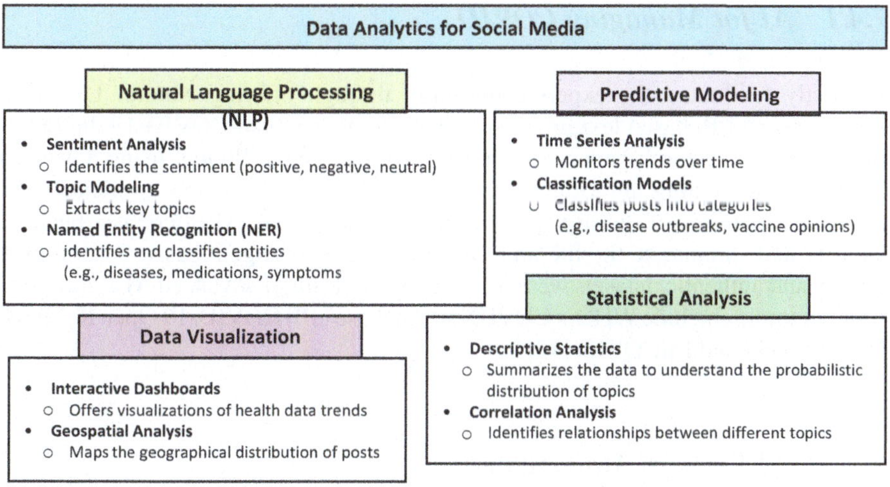

Fig. 7.4 Data science techniques for social media analytics

It is also important to note that despite having numerous advantages for using social media to infer population health trends, there are also various challenges. For example, there could be misinformation as anyone can post about anything on the social media, which could often lead to false interpretation about disease outbreaks, risk factors, unavailability of medical resources, etc. There are always privacy concerns which may restrict users from sharing their complete information on social media; this on one hand will protect the user's confidentiality, but on the other hand, may restrict the use of analytics as the lack of information may create hurdles for population health assessment. Moreover, social media is known to cause mental health issues due to creating anxiety about various social issues; this trend could also lead to false interpretations of population mental health inferred by data analytics. There are also legal, ethical and professional concerns about using social media for posting health-related information. All these challenges will affect the potential of data analytics for true identification of population health trends and risks.

7.4 Artificial Intelligence for Population Health Management

Artificial intelligence tools such as ML and DL algorithms have introduced novel applications in the domain of healthcare. The data generated from the lower levels of IoT-DS-AI nexus is finally fed into AI for developing preventive measures targeting improving population health outcomes. Most of the time, the applications of AI in healthcare with a focus on individual health can also be scaled to incorporate the public health. In this section, we present some of the approaches that deployed AI for managing population health:

7.4.1 AI for Managing COVID

AI firstly facilitated the expert community through offering Natural Language Processing (NLP) based text processing. During the years of COVID-19, hundreds of reports and research papers were published every day. Without using advanced AI based text mining algorithms, it could not have been possible to identify the trends and patterns of disease spread, high risk areas, etc. AI offers assistance to identify and summarize the literature for the experts on urgent basis. Several high quality and authentic datasets were developed as a result of advanced AI algorithms; some examples include WHO's COVID-19 database [10] COVID-19 Open Research Data Set [11] and LitCOVID [12].

7.4.2 AI for Staff Management

The data from the IoT and DS algorithms is fed into AI tools for managing the hospital staff, particularly doctors and nurses. AI algorithms can optimize shift scheduling by considering various factors such as staff availability, qualifications, and patient needs, ensuring adequate coverage while minimizing overtime and reducing burnout. AI also plays an important role in the modern workforce allocation systems through skill matching; this also ensures the retention and engagement of employees. As previously mentioned, IoT devices and data analytics algorithms help to streamline the patient flows; AI is next in the nexus and facilitates predicting the patient flows, which in turn help to manage the shift hours and allocate resources to wards and hospitals according to the expected workload.

Various innovative proposals have been made for using AI for healthcare staff monitoring. A simple algorithm SVM could be used for monitoring drowsiness in the nursing staff [13]. Again, IoT and ambient sensors can be used to identify the work habits, and physiological indications of employees, which are used to detect sleepiness using SVM that has been trained over extensive sleep dataset. Subsequently alerts can be generated for the relevant employee and their team leads to reduce the chances of accidents. This would not only reduce the medical errors but would also assist the authorities to review and evaluate their working hours/staff shifts policies. Similarly, AI based tools and simulators have been developed for offering trainings to the staff, which also improves the quality of services they offer.

AI algorithms also provide various insight about the performance analysis of workforce, as well as predictions about the turnover rate. The top performers in each hospital can quickly be identified by running the AI algorithms that work on various performance related metrics of employee; some metric would be number of errors made, number of absences, average response time for patient requests, patient satisfaction rates, number of tasks completed, team collaboration, etc. Hence, use of AI for workforce management at the hospitals facilitates the state decision making about new hirings in the sector, relocation of the existing staff, required number of new medical graduates, etc. Since the availability and retention of healthcare staff has a direct influence over quality of care extended to the patients, AI serves the governments for effective human resource planning.

7.4.3 AI for Health Disaster Detection

Natural disasters are often associated with healthcare crises for affected states. AI models assist to predict these disasters through assessing the data received from various sources such as IoT sensors. Algorithms of logistic regression, KNN, SVM and decision tree can predict earthquakes and their severity for specific regions; neural networks can be trained to predict floods; random forest can be used to predict typhoons. Most of these predictions can be made on low computing intensive edge devices which further adds to the cost-effectiveness of using technology for disaster monitoring [14]. All these computations are then transmitted to central state dashboards to facilitate analysis about the impact of disaster, observation of trends, and planning for resource allocation to manage the public health emergencies.

7.4.4 AI Integration with Social Media

Big data generated from social media is also analyzed by AI algorithms for identifying various aspects of population health. The hierarchy of public health actions taken with the help of AI applied on social media data has been presented in Fig. 7.5:

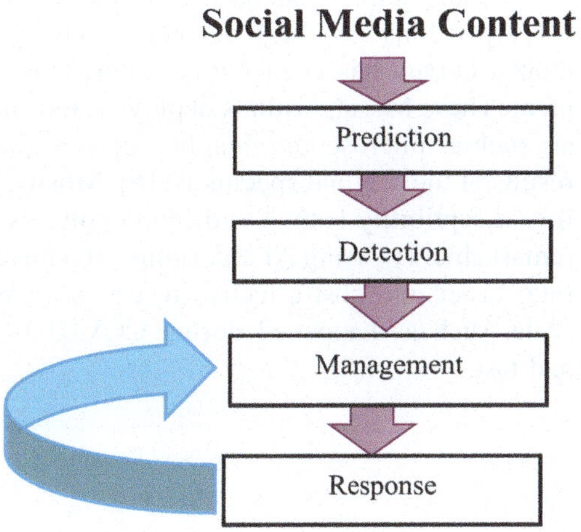

Fig. 7.5 Flow of actions by AI algorithms for social media analytics

AI algorithms ranging from simple to complex, all can be applied for predicting and detecting various health issues and public perceptions/concerns about them. For example, DL models are widely used for interpreting the datasets generated by social media. DL model has been developed for assessing the impact of COVID on population's mental health [15]; similar models have been proposed for early detection of disaster achieved through aggregating data from millions of social media accounts; furthermore, ML algorithms can also provide insight into disaster by quickly analyzing the camera feeds received from social media account and public cameras. Clearly, the early detection helps the authorities to plan efficient allocation of resources which improves the chances of minimizing casualties.

As shown in Fig. 7.5, the AI tools, using social media data can predict the upcoming health disaster or concerns of population. These algorithms could also detect the occurrence of disasters quicker as compared to the conventional methods. The data received from GPS sensors in integration with social media posts facilitate to identify the pin-point location of disaster. Once detected, the decision support systems fueled by AI algorithms and tools such as ChatGPT can offer advise to the policymakers for efficient strategies based on the learning from best global practices. Furthermore, the impact of the policies implemented can also be evaluated using social media feed again. Interestingly, the policymakers also get an opportunity to even modify their policies with the help of social media analytics and AI as also illustrated by Fig. 7.5.

7.4.5 AI for Large-Scale Lab Diagnostics

The modern healthcare systems rely largely on the labs and other assessment. All the processes of diagnosing, treating and managing the diseases are influenced by the quality of lab tests. AI clearly surpasses human understanding and interpretation of lab samples mainly due to learning from millions of data points. Several ML algorithms have been developed and tested for detecting microorganisms and their accuracy has been found comparable with the conventional testing equipment. These ML algorithms deploy various modern techniques to develop diagnosis such as microscopic imaging, gene sequencing and metagenomic sequencing results of the original specimen [16]. Mostly, the use of AI has been recommended for susceptibility testing and blood cultures as accuracy in these areas has been remarkable. By using AI algorithms, the governments get benefits of having accurate, faster and cost-effective test results. When conducting tests on a massive scale, such as happened during COVID-19, AI can make the process efficient and fast.

7.5 Critical Factors for Using Technology for Population Health Surveillance and Resource Optimization

As discussed in this chapter, the integration of IoT, Data Science (DS), and Artificial Intelligence (AI) offers transformative potential for population health surveillance and healthcare resource optimization. These technologies, provide real-time, comprehensive insights into public health trends, emerging health threats, and healthcare resource usage. In this section, we present some of the critical factors which must be taken care of, while deploying these technologies.

7.5.1 Data Collection and Integration

The role of IoT devices is fundamental to the IoT-DS-AI nexus. The deployment of wearable and/or ambient IoT devices is crucial for gathering diverse health-related data. These devices enable continuous and remote monitoring of individuals' health metrics, such as heart rate, blood pressure, and air quality, which provides the basis of population health analytics and risk predictions. Once the data is obtained, next phase is of data integration, which is also a crucial requirement for population health assessment. Data from diverse sources must be integrated including those generated by IoT devices, electronic health records (EHRs), social media, and public health databases.

7.5.2 Ensuring Quality of Data

It is essential to ensure the quality, reliability, accuracy and precision of the IoT devices at the lowest tier of IoT-DS-AI nexus, as it would govern the entire process of population health management. In case data sensed and transmitted by IoT devices is inaccurate, all the reliability of decision-making process may be compromised. It is also important to deploy effective data science methodologies to clean and preprocess the vast amounts of data collected, removing noise and addressing inconsistencies.

7.5.3 Advanced Analytics and Predictive Modeling

Once the cleaned data is available, advanced ML and DL techniques are used for analyzing large datasets and identifying patterns, trends, and anomalies. Predictive modeling helps in forecasting disease outbreaks, identifying at-risk populations, and optimizing resource allocation. It is critical to identify and deploy the most suitable ML/DL models to be able to reach the correct population health inferences. In this context, the capabilities and limitations of various algorithms must be taken care of.

7.5.4 Interoperability and Standardization

As we have seen, each layer of the IoT-DS-AI nexus makes use of a large number of devices and software platforms, the heterogeneity of these platforms makes it a challenge to exchange the information between them. It is vital to developing interoperable systems that can communicate and share data efficiently, for a comprehensive population health surveillance. In this regard, standardization would facilitate the seamless exchange and utilization of data across various platforms.

7.5.5 User Adoption and Training

For both the aspects of population health surveillance and healthcare resource optimization, it is mandatory that patients and healthcare professionals agree to use the required hardware/software/mobile apps, etc. Resistance to change and the learning curve associated with new technologies must be mitigated through comprehensive training programs, for both the sectors of patients and professionals. For patients, engaging the public and raising awareness about the benefits of IoT and data analytics for health surveillance can enhance user adoption and participation. On the other hand, training healthcare professionals to effectively use IoT devices and interpret data analytics is essential for achieving efficient population health surveillance and resource optimization.

7.5.6 Policy and Regulation

There is still a lack of policies, laws and regulations that govern the use of computing and communication technologies for individual and population health management. Regulations that address data privacy, security, and ethical considerations need to be developed and implemented. Government and institutional support through policies that promote the adoption of these technologies is crucial to achieve their full potential in the domain of public health.

7.5.7 *Privacy and Security*

When particularly managing individual or population health using technology, the focus is mostly on generating and sharing human subject data. In the past, the patient history was managed on paper files and also the survey forms were usually collected on paper; hence, there was much lesser probability of sensitive information leakage as compared to today. Therefore, robust data privacy measures, including anonymization and encryption, must be implemented to safeguard sensitive information.

In addition, we not only have to be cautious for the human element, but also for the IT infrastructure security. It is critical to ensure the security of IoT devices, cloud servers and data analytics platforms to sustain the public trust on technology. Failing to do so will lead to limited or no deployment of IoT-AI-DS nexus for individual as well as population health surveillance.

References

1. WHO EMRO I Public health surveillance I Health topics. Accessed 02 Aug 2024. [Online]. Available: https://www.emro.who.int/health-topics/public-health-surveillance/index.html
2. K.S. Sahu, S.E. Majowicz, J.A. Dubin, P.P. Morita, NextGen public health surveillance and the Internet of Things (IoT). Front. Public Health **9** (2021). https://doi.org/10.3389/fpubh.2021.756675
3. Y.J. Tseng, K.L. Olson, D. Bloch, K.D. Mandl, Smart thermometer-based participatory surveillance to discern the role of children in household viral transmission during the COVID-19 pandemic. JAMA Netw. Open **6**(6) (2023). https://doi.org/10.1001/jamanetworkopen.2023.16190
4. S.D. Chamberlain, I. Singh, C. Ariza, A. Daitch, P. Philips, B.D. Dalziel, Real-time detection of COVID-19 epicenters within the United States using a network of smart thermometers. medRxiv (2020). https://doi.org/10.1101/2020.04.06.20039909
5. R.Z. Wan-Chik, N.S.S.B. Zamri, S.S.B. Hasbullah, Technology application in airports reopening and operations recovery due to COVID-19 pandemic, in *Technology Application in Aviation, Tourism and Hospitality: Recent Developments and Emerging Issues*, (2022). https://doi.org/10.1007/978-981-19-6619-4_11
6. A. Roy, F.H. Kumbhar, H.S. Dhillon, N. Saxena, S.Y. Shin, S. Singh, Efficient monitoring and contact tracing for COVID-19: A smart IoT-based framework. IEEE Internet Things Mag. **3**(3) (2020). https://doi.org/10.1109/IOTM.0001.2000145
7. Z. Wang et al., From personalized medicine to population health: A survey of mHealth sensing techniques. IEEE Internet Things J. (2022). https://doi.org/10.1109/JIOT.2022.3161046
8. J. Malathi, K.R. Kusha, S. Isaac, A. Ramesh, M. Rajendiran, S. Boopathi, *IoT-Enabled Remote Patient Monitoring for Chronic Disease Management and Cost Savings: Transforming Healthcare* (2024. https://services.igi-global.com/resolvedoi/resolve.aspx?doi=10.4018/978-1-6684-6361-1.ch014), pp. 371–388. https://doi.org/10.4018/978-1-6684-6361-1.CH014
9. S. Kanchan, A. Gaidhane, Social media role and its impact on public health: A narrative review. Cureus (2023). https://doi.org/10.7759/cureus.33737
10. Coronavirus (COVID-19) Cases and Deaths—WHO-COVID-19-global-data.csv—Humanitarian Data Exchange. Accessed 02 Aug 2024. [Online]. Available: https://data.humdata.org/dataset/coronavirus-covid-19-cases-and-deaths/resource/2ac6c3c0-76fa-4486-9ad0-9aa9e253b78d

11. COVID-19 Open Research Dataset (CORD-19). https://doi.org/10.5281/ZENODO.3731937
12. E. Zhang, N. Gupta, R. Nogueira, K. Cho, J. Lin, Rapidly deploying a neural search engine for the COVID-19 open research dataset, in *Proceedings of the Annual Meeting of the Association for Computational Linguistics*, (2020)
13. B.J. Ganesh, P. Vijayan, V. Vaidehi, S. Murugan, R. Meenakshi, M. Rajmohan, SVM-based predictive modeling of drowsiness in hospital staff for occupational safety solution via IoT infrastructure, in *2024 2nd International Conference on Computer, Communication and Control, IC4 2024*, (2024). https://doi.org/10.1109/IC457434.2024.10486429
14. M. Aboualola, K. Abualsaud, T. Khattab, N. Zorba, H.S. Hassanein, Edge technologies for disaster management: A survey of social media and artificial intelligence integration. IEEE Access **11** (2023). https://doi.org/10.1109/ACCESS.2023.3293035
15. M.H. Al Banna et al., A hybrid deep learning model to predict the impact of COVID-19 on mental health from social media big data. IEEE Access **11** (2023). https://doi.org/10.1109/ACCESS.2023.3293857
16. S.A. Alowais et al., Revolutionizing healthcare: The role of artificial intelligence in clinical practice. BMC Med. Educ. (2023). https://doi.org/10.1186/s12909-023-04698-z

Chapter 8
The Way Forward

8.1 Challenges

8.1.1 Outdated Infrastructure

The outdated computing infrastructure of medical facilities causes one of the major hurdles in the deployment of IoT for numerous applications. Since the core of IoT integration exists in data collection, processing and analytics, the computing facilities available should be advanced enough to accommodate these needs. Unfortunately, many medical facilities still rely on legacy systems that lack the capacity to handle the vast amounts of data generated by IoT devices. This limitation not only hampers the efficiency of data processing but also affects the real-time analysis and decision-making crucial for patient care.

8.1.2 Volume of Generated Data

Integrating IoT solutions within the healthcare domain creates tremendous amount of data. The typical IoT applications for the hospitals involve monitoring the hospitalized and at-home, integration with Electronic Health Records, monitoring the resources, monitoring the staff, monitoring/managing the medical equipment and improve the overall operations such as reducing the waiting time for Emergency Room or reducing the electricity consumption [2]. All of these processes generate massive amounts of data, which must be realized by all the stakeholders. The hospitals and other relevant facilities should have secure space available for storing the data, either online or offline. In addition to the capacity of storing and processing data, the hospitals also need to develop/implement efficient policies for secured access to patients' data. In case the organizations are not prepared for managing the

S. Siddiqui et al., *Connected Health Insights for Sustainable Development*,
https://doi.org/10.1007/978-3-031-81433-4_8

challenges such as data ownership, access rights, authorization and accountability, there could be serious obstacles caused for attaining the full potential of health IoT systems.

8.1.3 Increased Vulnerabilities

Connecting massive number of IoT devices into the healthcare sphere simply means offering more points of intrusion to the attackers. Health IoT devices provide a good opportunity to hackers, not only for breaching into the hospital's IT infrastructure but also to alter the medical equipment/apps to send altered medical information; hence the use IoT does not only risks hospital's infrastructure, but also the life and well-being of patients. There is a serious lack of standards for the IoT equipment often used in healthcare due to the diversity of manufacturers and platforms; this further complicates the enforcement of robust security measures.

8.1.4 Confidentiality and Privacy

As discussed throughout the book, the users of healthcare technology are required to provide details about their present and past medical history, family, lifestyle etc. For the innovative applications such as population health surveillance requires more and more personal data. Sharing this information makes the users prone to breaches and attacks. People are always doubtful about unauthorized access which could happen due to vulnerabilities in IoT devices or network security. Also, patients may have limited control over their data once its collected and shared among various systems as there is still a lack of framework for data sharing and data ownership; there is also no specific consent-management techniques for digital patient data, that used to be a norm for older paper-based survey forms. Modern data integration also creates challenges for assuring confidentiality and privacy because even after anonymization, it is possible that personal identities are revealed due to combining multiple data sources. Similarly, people are increasingly becoming aware of the data analytics and AI biases which could lead to discriminations in healthcare decision for them.

8.1.5 User Adoption

One of the major challenges in implementing health IoT solutions is the need for extensive training for healthcare professionals. Doctors, nurses, administrative staff, and other healthcare workers must learn to use new IoT technologies effectively, which can be time-consuming and costly. Resistance to change is common, as many professionals may be skeptical about the reliability of automated systems for critical diagnostics and treatment decisions. The steep learning curve associated with these advanced technologies can further hinder adoption, as healthcare workers might find it difficult to integrate new workflows into their established routines. Additionally, patients often struggle with understanding and using personal IoT health devices, which can lead to incorrect data collection and reduced effectiveness of these technologies. Particularly, due to the existing digital divide in the developing countries, it would be a challenge to convince people to put IoT devices to a regular usage [3]. Since both the healthcare professionals and patients in these regions may lack the necessary skills and resources to effectively utilize IoT technologies, it would be even tougher to deploy them.

8.2 Managing the Challenges

The users need to be first convinced about the expected benefit of health IoT systems, and subsequently basic trainings must be offered to reduce the hesitation with the use of technology/apps. Healthcare professionals need to be trained to use new IoT technologies effectively. This includes not only doctors but also nurses, administrative staff, and other healthcare workers who interact with IoT systems. Resistance to change and the learning curve associated with new technologies can impede the adoption of IoT solutions. Doctors may be hesitant to rely on automated systems for critical diagnostics and treatment decisions, while nurses and other staff might find the new workflows disruptive and challenging to integrate into their daily routines. Moreover, patients also need to be educated on how to use personal IoT health devices accurately to ensure they benefit from these technologies. Comprehensive training programs and ongoing support are essential to ensure all users feel confident and proficient in using IoT technologies, which is crucial for the successful implementation and maximization of IoT benefits in healthcare settings. Some of the major recommendations offered as a result of in-depth analysis presented in this book follows next:

8.2.1 Reliability and Performance

The core requirement of the development and implementation of ambitious deployment of IoT-DS-AI nexus is to ensure its reliability and satisfactory performance at various levels of hierarchy. To begin with, a scalable and fault-tolerant architecture must be designed to store and process large volumes of data. Efficient computing and communication strategies must be adopted as per the requirements; for example, distributed computing should be used for reducing latency and managing the real-time processing, such as use of fog, edge and cloud computing. To maintain the functionality and reduce downtime, redundant systems should also be developed.

Since the healthcare decision making is largely governed by data analytics and AI algorithms in the IoT-DS-AI nexus, it is crucial to ensure the quality and authenticity of data. High-quality data collection, preprocessing, and cleaning must be practiced to improve the reliability of AI models and DS analyses. Also, robust data integration frameworks should be adopted to seamlessly combine data from various IoT devices and sources. Before any healthcare technology is implemented, significant level of testing and validation should be done to ensure satisfactory operation from end-to-end. Extensive testing, including unit tests, integration tests, and system tests, should be performed to ensure each component functions correctly. Similarly, performance of AI models should be validated against real-world data to ensure accuracy, reliability, and relevance.

Once tested and implemented, continuous monitoring and regular audits of these systems should follow. Since the new vulnerabilities emerge every day, it is crucial to ensure safety of these systems, as individual as well as population health could be at stake. For the entire system including IoT devices, DS models and AI algorithms, regular audits should be performed to detect and address issues promptly. Moreover, as discussed previously in Chap. 3, predictive maintenance should be practiced to further improve the reliability of system.

8.2.2 Security, Privacy, Ethics and Law

It has been universally accepted that there is a need to develop and implement standards, regulations and laws for governing the uses of computing and communication technologies for the healthcare domain. Some actions have been taken in this regard; for example, a digital psychiatry task force has been formulated by American Psychiatric Association (APA) for monitoring and evaluating the technology and particularly AI solutions being used for mental health assessment and therapies. Such taskforces will be responsible for assessing the technology solution for their safety, efficacy, tolerability in addition to the usual evaluation of efficiency/quality of offered services. Similarly, standards for evaluation of technology tools have also been developed. APA has developed an App Evaluation Model called App Advisor which could provide assistance to the users in choosing the health apps. This model has also been replicated and used by other companies such as Division of Digital Psychiatry and BIDMC at Harvard University App Evaluation [4]. It is hence, expected that the healthcare solutions will be standardized soon.

There are various measures adopted by healthcare users and authorities to maintain security, privacy and ethics. First and foremost, the hospitals and other stakeholders have to ensure adherence to the available standards and regulations such as HIPAA (Health Insurance Portability and Accountability Act), GDPR (General Data Protection Regulation); this measure guarantees that health data is handled in a legally compliant and secure manner. Also, there are regular security audits and compliance checks which help to identify and address potential security weaknesses in the system. Secondly, there are technical measures such as encryption; it is ensured that all data transferred or stored remains protected by preventing unauthorized access. Strict access controls have to be implemented; most commonly role-based access controls or multi-factor authentication methods are used. Another common method of ensuring patient privacy is anonymization of patient data; all such information that can lead to identifying the patients is removed before analyzing the data or sharing it with third parties. Moreover, data minimization is also an important technique which refers to restricting to collecting only that data which is crucial.

8.2.3 Interoperability

Adopting the standards and legal framework is the major approach to ensure interoperability between the systems within each level and between the levels of IoT-DS-AI nexus. Similar communication protocols (such as MQTT, CoAP, and HTTP/HTTPS for IoT devices) must be used by different manufacturers, and wherever needs, APIs and middleware should be used for creating a hub between multiple products. For the efficient transmission and processing of data between cross-systems, common data models and ontologies should be used to represent healthcare data, such as SNOMED CT and LOINC. Moreover, data transformation and normalization processes should also be developed and implemented. Another best health industry-wide practice could be to develop interoperability frameworks that support multiple protocols and standards to act as a bridge between IoT, AI, and DS systems; for example, Service-Oriented Architecture (SOA) principles can be used to design systems.

It is to be noted that maintaining interoperability will also in turn facilitate the aspects of flexibility and scalability. The population health systems are expected to enhance in the coming future, and ensuring that new systems can continue to be the part of initially developed infrastructure is the key to success for individual and population health management.

8.2.4 User Training and Support

Despite increasing deployment of technical solutions in the domain of healthcare, there still remain significant user resistance to adopt these. Some of these reasons include the fear of technology, lack of digital literacy and concerns about privacy and security. For the goal of achieving good health for all, it is mandatory that users accept and adopt the technology as they are the major stakeholders and mostly, also the first point of data entry. Trainings must be provided to healthcare staff to effectively use and manage IoT, DS, and AI systems. Throughout the lifecycle of IoT-DS-AI nexus, comprehensive technical support must be offered to the hospital staff to address any issues that arise. Likewise, awareness campaigns and trainings should be developed for the public in order to convince them to use and appreciate the technology.

References

1. T. Shaik et al., Remote patient monitoring using artificial intelligence: Current state, applications, and challenges. Wiley Interdiscip. Rev.: Data Min. Knowl. Discov. **2023**, e1485 (2023). https://doi.org/10.1002/widm.1485
2. K.H. Almotairi, Application of internet of things in healthcare domain. J. Umm Al-Qura Univ. Eng. Archit. **14**(1) (2023). https://doi.org/10.1007/s43995-022-00008-8
3. J.A. Hoyos Muñoz, D. Cardona Valencia, Trends and challenges of digital divide and digital inclusion: A bibliometric analysis. J. Inf. Sci. (2023). https://doi.org/10.1177/01655515221148366
4. AI is changing every aspect of psychology. Here's what to watch for. Accessed 03 Aug 2024. [Online]. Available: https://www.apa.org/monitor/2023/07/psychology-embracing-ai

The manufacturer's authorised representative in the EU is Springer Nature Customer Service Centre GmbH, Europaplatz 3, 69115 Heidelberg, Germany. If you have any concerns regarding our products, please contact ProductSafety@springernature.com

Printed and bound by CPI Group (UK) Ltd, Croydon, CR0 4YY
30/09/2026
02225575-0015